Touch + Stretch

Dedication

In writing this book I am only too aware of
the number of people who have taught me
the things that you will find in my pages.
There are, of course, dozens of such people,
some contributing much knowledge, some
no more than a small but useful tip.
"In progressing, we stand on the shoulders
of giants," said someone: it is to all my giants
that this book is dedicated.

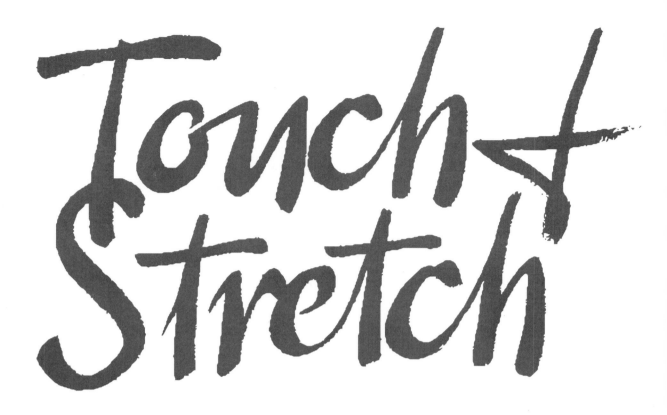

Touch + Stretch

Carolan Evans

MACKENZIE

Publisher's note: This book includes therapeutic massage instructions for the reader to follow. However, not all massage therapies are designed for all individuals. Before starting these or any other massage or exercise programmes you may wish to consult your doctor for advice.

First published in Great Britain in 1991 by
Mackenzie Publishing Limited
178 Royal College Street, London NW1 0PS

Concept, design and production by
Terry Allen

Editorial **Chris Gosselin**

Photography **Chris Sowe**

A catalogue record for this book is available from the British Library

ISBN 0- 951 6355 1 4

Typeset by Terry Allen Design Consultants Limited, London

Reproduction by P R Service Graphique Paris

Computer generated film by Keene Engraving

Printed and bound in Great Britain by Butler & Tanner Ltd, Frome and London

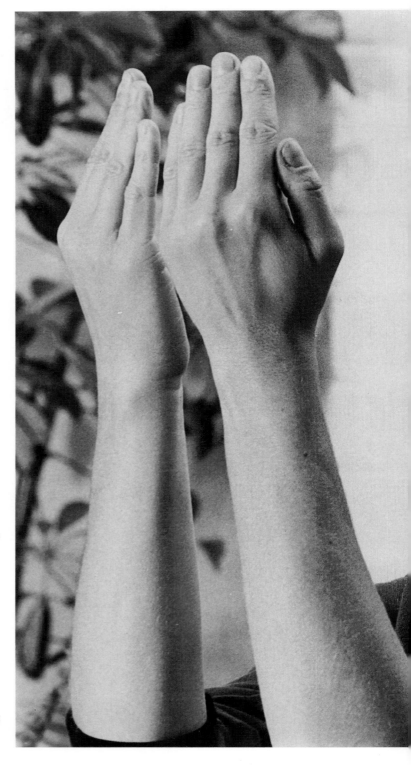

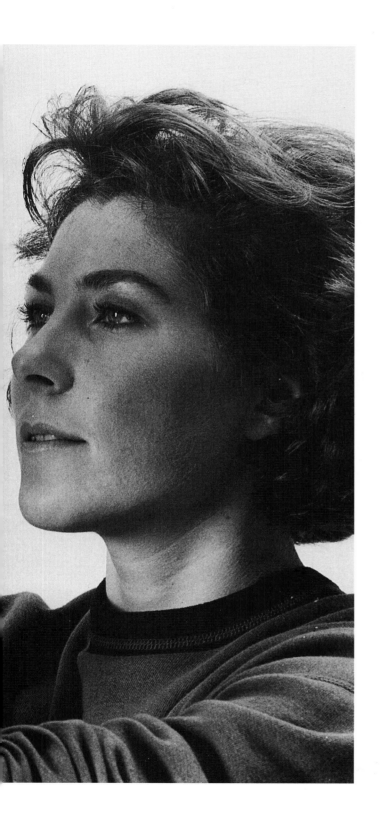

CONTENTS

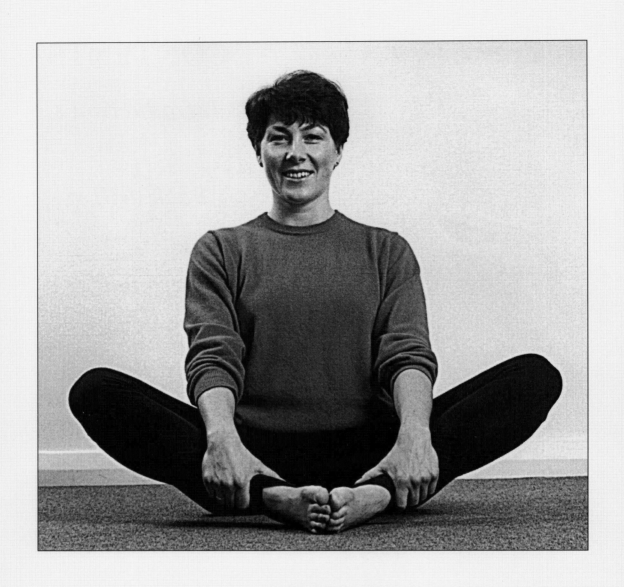

Introduction

Let self massage and stretching balance
the stresses in your life

Maintaining a healthy body

In our everyday activities, we do not often think of the incredibly complex way our minds and bodies interact to produce movement. We take care of our cars and household appliances, yet seldom think of the mechanisms that lie within us until something goes wrong.

However, we *do* sometimes notice the signals our bodies transmit to us. When we have to remain seated for a time, we become aware of a need to stretch our legs and get a breath of fresh air. If our head aches or we hurt ourselves, we instinctively use our hands to ease the pain. Touching and stretching are natural extensions of our instinctive response to body signals. They help us to get to know our body's structure and to feel comfortable within our skin. Also, as an added bonus, much disease can be prevented when we become more aware of the signs and signals our body sends out and react quickly to them.

Muscle power -- movement and tension

The skeleton is the basic frame or scaffolding of the body structure. There are minor variations from person to person, but a row of skeletons hung up would all look pretty much the same -- and all would be *straight*. When we are balanced, our bones line up to support the weight of the body: this is why we talk of hips and knees as 'weight-bearing joints'.

Muscles at work

What makes each of us an individual is muscle. Muscles are the movers of the body and they are fixed to the bones by tendons, whilst ligaments hold the joints together.

Muscles work in pairs: one contracts to move a part of the body, whilst its partner contracts to reverse the movement.

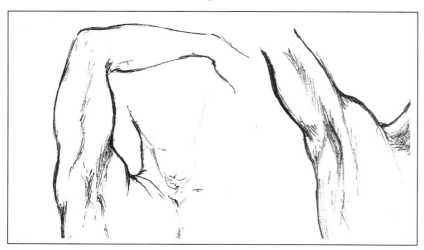

Most people can readily see the biceps muscle in the front of the upper arm when they flex the arm at the elbow. To return the arm to a straight position, the triceps muscle at the back of the arm contracts and the biceps relaxes.

Learning to move freely

Although many of our movements seem instinctive, most have had to be learnt and built into a repertoire that makes us move in our own individual way, including areas of free-flowing and graceful movement, areas of stiffness and areas of dexterity and skill.

For effective movement a certain amount of 'tone' is necessary in the muscles, but if that tone is excessive it develops into tension. At first this tension is not registered by the brain and so can build up, pulling the body out of balance because it usually affects one muscle to a greater extent than its partner. The imbalance can become habitual, strain being passed on through the joints, which become stiff, limiting our range of movement.

Since the process of creating stiffness and tension in the body is partly emotional and partly physical, we must employ both emotional and physical methods to oppose that process and release the stresses that have been built up.

Letting go of your tensions

When you massage your own body, you are able to be very specific in finding the precise area of tension and determining the exact amount of pressure needed to relieve it. Nevertheless, you need to remember that you are both the active *and* the passive partner; you are both giving the massage and receiving it. As a result, total relaxation is not always too easy to achieve. For this reason, use as many aids to relaxation as you can (see Chapter 1). Let your hands really explore and feel your body in a new way. Close your eyes and experience the difference in your awareness of touch: become aware at first of the reluctance of your body to 'let go'.

We often move tension from one area to another -- largely because the body has not yet learned how to get rid of tension completely -- so you will also learn in this book how to discover your own patterns of tension and release.

The strokes illustrated form the basis for the whole repertoire of massage. Once you know the rules, you can be creative within the system and devise your own unique style to help yourself and also your friends and family. The sequence of strokes described below applies to whatever part of the body is being massaged.

Effleurage

Begin with the light stroking movements known as effleurage. The movements are just like stroking a pet animal, hands held relaxed and moulding themselves to the shape of your body.

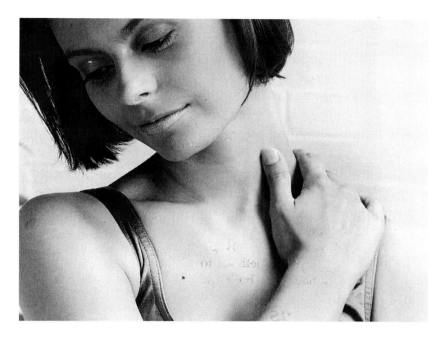

Effleurage is used to spread oil if you are using it, to bring awareness to the area being worked, to relax it and encourage the circulation of blood and lymph. These circulatory systems are vital to nourish the tissues and to clear toxins.

Kneading /petrissage

Follow effleurage with kneading movements. These use the whole hand in the manner of kneading dough and are designed to penetrate deeper into the muscle tissue. Petrissage movements are done with the balls of fingers or thumbs making pressures towards the bone.

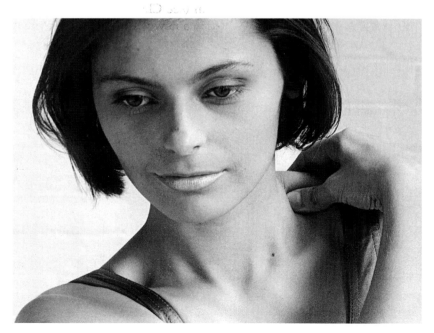

When the bulk of the muscle is warmed up and soft, use small circular pressures into the areas of tension. These circular friction movements, carried out with thumbs, fingers or the heel of the hand are used to release localised areas of tension within the muscle.

Tapotement

If the muscles do not relax and soften during the kneading, then petrissage is inappropriate and tapping and rapping movements, generally known as tapotement, should be used first. These include small hitting movements, such as taps, slaps and rapping with a loosely-closed fist, or 'piano playing' with the fingers.

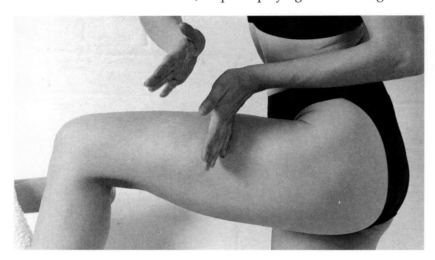

Tapotement should be done with hands and wrists relaxed, otherwise the effect will be painful. Once the muscle has let go, proceed with petrissage and finish with some more effleurage movements to soothe the area and encourage the dispersal of toxins through the lymphatic circulation.

Stretching for maximum effect

Your body has mechanisms to protect itself from extremes of movement, so that it can maintain stability. So, when stretching, move to the point of mild discomfort -- but not pain! As you hold the position, imagine that you are able to breathe through the part of you that feels tight or tense. Visualise the movement you would like to make and gently *allow* it to happen. You should therefore synchronise your outbreath with further gentle movement into the stretch. Keep these further movements gentle: *never* bounce into the stretch.

Breathing and imagination

There is no 'correct' way of breathing, different breathing patterns being appropriate to different activities. Sometimes, however when we are concentrating, we hold our breath, and this is counter-productive to good touch-and-stretch practices. Concentration on breathing has an effect on the mind, a fact used in meditation techniques; the mind has in turn a powerful effect on the body, and use of your imagination in creating visualisations can make movement and relaxation very much more effective.

The term 'visualisation' can seem a little daunting to people who believe that they cannot visualise. However, everyone has a vivid imagination, so try to become aware of the cycle of your breath and imagine the good effects the air you breathe in is having when it reaches the parts of the body you are working on. Picture to yourself the benefits of the work you are doing: you will be surprised how powerful this technique is in maximising the benefits involved.

Maybe you would like a neck as graceful as a swan, or a spine as lithe as an acrobat's? With practice and a little imagination to help you, all things are possible!

How long should your sessions take?

Since everyone is different, both in their ability to let go and relax and on the time they have for themselves alone, it is difficult to make rules. As a general guideline, however, each of the massage strokes described in this book should be performed 4-6 times at least, whilst the stretches should be held for a minimum of 30 seconds each. For many of us, relaxation and visualisation are not easy, and it takes a certain amount of commitment to the practice before the real benefits manifest. When I was learning a particular technique, the instructor used to say that to practise 5 minutes a day was good, 10 minutes was very good and 15 minutes excellent -- in other words, whatever time you think you can spare will be beneficial. When you start, focussing your attention for even two minutes can seem a very long time, but you will soon find you can extend this period and begin to enjoy the whole experience.

Using this book effectively

For quick reference, Touch and Stretch is divided into sections covering different areas of your body so that you can concentrate on the sequences for whichever area is in need of attention. However, because the body is a complex structure of interrelated parts, we cannot really treat one area as an isolated unit. While using the book, try to keep a holistic (whole body) approach in mind, and become aware of the way different areas of your body interact. For example, working on tense neck and shoulder muscles can relieve a headache and also free areas of your upper back and chest, making breathing easier.

Always start with the massage sequence to loosen muscles and increase circulation in the area affected. Then move on to your stretches, which use the body's own weight to stretch the muscles further and free the joints. With both the massage and the stretch movements, always follow a routine of 'do -- stop -- feel the result'.

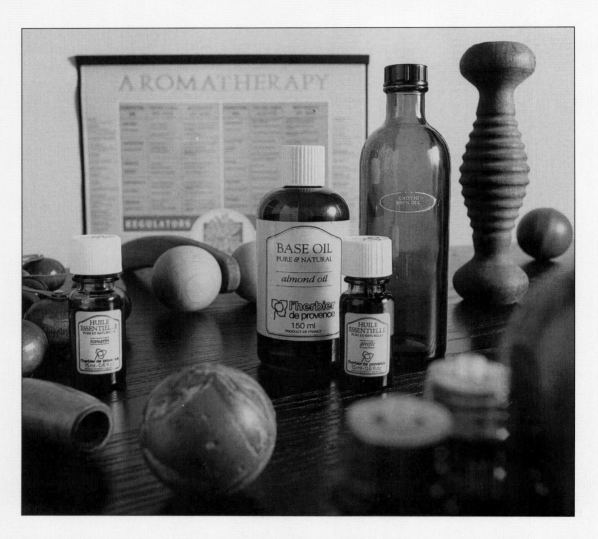

1
Pack drill

*For effective stretching, equipment is unnecessary.
For massage, you need very little more than your
bare hands and a few essential oils.*

Getting down to essentials

The most essential parts of your equipment are your own body and hands, so keeping the joints of your hands and fingers strong and supple is vital to successful massage and will also ensure that they maintain maximum movement throughout later life. Take a few minutes to exercise your hands, beginning by rubbing them together to encourage circulation. Then . . .

Steeple your fingers and press them hard together to increase their strength. Flick out the fingers one by one.

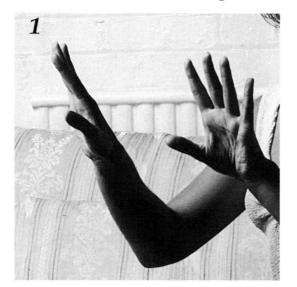
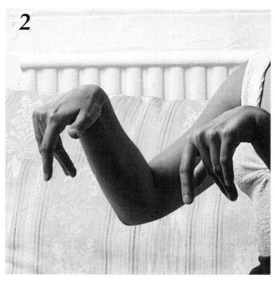

1 and **2** Perform wrist circles clockwise and anti-clockwise

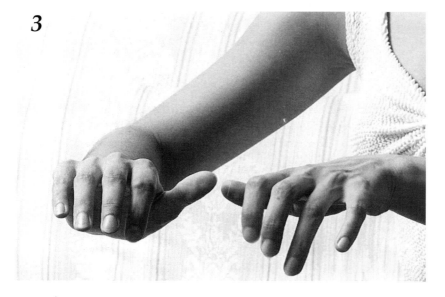

3 Play an imaginary piano to get all the fingers working.

Finding the right medium

Think next about the massage itself and how you want it to feel. Massage can be done through clothing, but it feels very much better, and is much more effective, when used directly on your skin with something to help the hands slide over the body without friction. In an emergency, however, you can use whatever comes to hand. For instance, if you have no talc, raid the kitchen for cornflour: if you prefer not to put oil on your skin, substitute a body lotion or even a hand cream. The best massage medium is oil. There are a number of good massage oils available, but it is much more fun, and cheaper, to mix your own and add a special fragrance to suit your mood.

Choosing oils with care

Bear in mind that the skin is able to absorb certain molecules, so make it a rule not to put anything on your skin that you wouldn't put into your mouth. Use vegetable oils, therefore, rather than mineral oils which clog the skin. Any good quality oil will do, though some are better than others: for instance, select an oil which has no odour of its own and add your own choice of perfume or essential oil.

If good penetration is required (as in aromatherapy, see below), use grapeseed, rapeseed or soya oils. Olive, sesame or avocado oils are wonderfully nourishing to the skin, but their own aroma can be a little off-putting, so when their properties are required they can be added in small quantities to other oils to enrich them. Sweet almond is a good choice because it can be used on both your body and your face.

Aromatherapy -- the natural way

Aromatherapy is an ancient art which utilises the aromatic oils of certain plants as an aid to lessening stress, to help relaxation, and for the therapeutic effects of the oils on the body's organs and systems, bringing them into harmony. These plant oils are known as 'essential oils' and work best when applied to the skin during massage. Because they have a directly beneficial effect on the skin as they penetrate into the body, essential oils are often used as beauty aids. However, it would be a mistake to regard this as their only function, as they are powerful therapeutic substances and care must be taken when using them.

What are essential oils?

Chemically, they are not oils at all. They are highly volatile aromatic hydrocarbons and it is thought that in the plants from which they are extracted they act like hormones to regulate systems and defend against infection. Nearly all essential oils are active against bacteria, and some are also active against viruses and fungal growth.

How does aromatherapy work?

Essential oils have an effect on the human body in two ways. Firstly, the volatile nature of the oil means that it is rapidly dispersed in the air and the aroma reaches the brain areas which perceive smell. These areas of the brain are also concerned with producing our moods, so the aroma directly influences our state of mind. Secondly, the essential oil molecules are small enough to penetrate through the skin, into the bloodstream and so to all the organs and systems of the body which they affect according to the properties of the oil used. Essential oils may be used purely as an inhalation for respiratory problems or to add fragrance to a room, or both modes of action may be employed by adding them to your bath. When essential oils are used in massage, however, their effects are amplified by the soothing pressure of the hands and fingers.

Buying and using essential oils

Pure essential oils are expensive, but because they are so concentrated they are economical to use, and if stored away from direct heat, light and moisture have a long shelf-life. If you only want to create a pleasant aroma, then buy a cheaper perfume oil which may be a second distillation of an essential oil or may be synthetic in origin. If you want the full benefit of a *pure* essential oil, then bear the following in mind:

• **The oil should not be a cheap substitute.**
If it feels oily or leaves a greasy mark on paper then it is already diluted and not a *pure essential oil.*

• **It should be sold in a coloured glass bottle -- preferably brown -- with a dropper closure. Never keep essential oils in plastic containers; they may interact with the plastic and lose their properties.**

• **With a few exceptions, essential oils must not be applied directly onto the skin. They must first be mixed and diluted with a 'carrier' oil. As a guide:**

> **Use 1 drop of essential oil for every 2 ml (roughly half a teaspoonful) of carrier oil.**

> **For a general massage, a total of 10 ml (two teaspoonsful) of carrier oil with 5 drops of essential oil should be sufficient.**

> **Certain oils such as lemongrass may irritate a sensitive skin and should be diluted even further.**

> **Although natural and safe when used correctly, certain oils should not be used during pregnancy. If you are pregnant, consult a specialist text on aromatherapy.**

Creating the right atmosphere

Now that you're ready to start, you must set the scene for maximum benefit. Although self-massage can be performed almost anywhere, it is much more beneficial if you have the time and space to spare, so now is the time to create a bit of that space for yourself, get away from your everyday routine, take the 'phone off the hook (relax -- if it's important, they'll ring again). Turn the lights down low or light candles to relax your eyes. Make sure you are comfortable and warm, especially if you are going to remove your clothes.

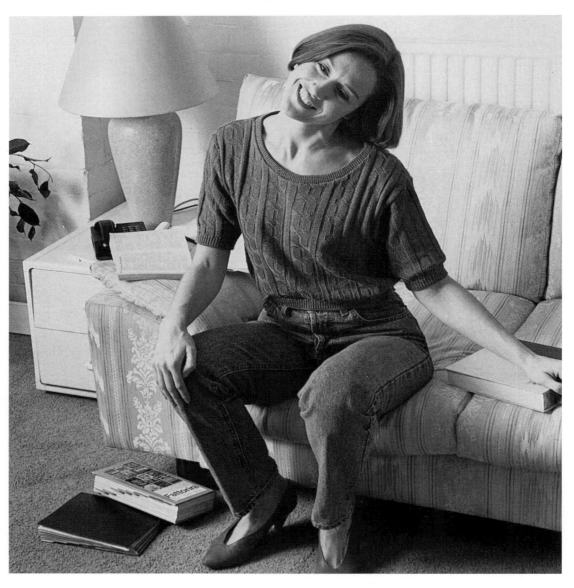

Mind and body at rest

Once your body is comfortable, start to let your mind relax and unwind. Remember those boring lessons at school when you doodled on your paper or daydreamed? That's exactly the state of mind to re-create now. Some people are able to reach this state through meditation, others find it helpful to listen to music, to watch fish in an aquarium, to sit and stroke a pet. Whatever your favourite technique, spend five minutes or so, allowing you to switch off and let your mind come to a restful state.

If you find relaxing difficult, then try taking a few really deep breaths and re-create in your imagination a place where you feel warm and relaxed. It may be a favourite walk or holiday place, but wherever you go in your imagination, try to make it as vivid an experience as possible, including sounds, smells and feelings. Keep that feeling as you begin to work on the tensions in your body using self-massage.

Commercial massage aids

These can be useful alternatives to using your hands and fingers, especially for those who have arthritic finger joints. There is a wide variety to choose from, including various types of rollers which can be used for the body and feet, massage mitts designed to be used with special products to eliminate cellulite, and vibrating pads with or without heat. Cheaper alternatives include a squash ball which can be used on the feet (see page 66) and a soft ball about the size of an orange which can be used for the body (see page 25).

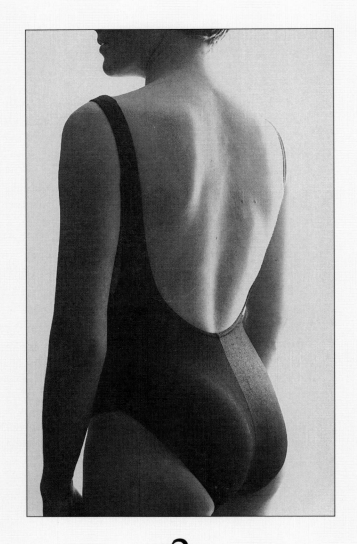

2
Back to basics

*Back problems are amongst the most common
complaints that fill doctors' surgeries...*

Most of our physical stresses and strains are felt in the back, and back problems are amongst the most common complaints that fill doctors' surgeries.

Back pain is often attributed to the fact that we stand upright against gravity. Look around and it's a fair bet that you won't see any truly upright bodies. Yet if you look at healthy small children you will see that we all start out straight, but as we get older and develop our own characteristic ways of holding ourselves and moving about, the natural upright becomes distorted. Within certain limits, we can all change our basic muscular shape and therefore affect the underlying skeletal structure. We can do this by strengthening the muscles which are weak compared with their opposites and by stretching and lengthening those which have been used too much.

The spinal cord

Ultimately everything is connected to the spinal bones or vertebrae. The spinal cord, which is the central communicator for the whole body, runs through a channel within the vertebrae. The nerves which connect to all the organs, systems and limbs emerge between these vertebrae. Keeping all this upright are the muscles of the back, balanced by those of the abdomen.

If you look at the body of a well-developed athlete or bodybuilder you will see that on either side of the spine there is a long band of muscle. Diagonally placed muscles run from below the shoulders down to the waist, giving the triangular look to the upper part of the body; round the shoulder and hip joints are groups of muscles which enable the complex movements of these joints. We all possess these muscle groups but in most of us they are less well defined. Because of the way muscles overlap, problems which are felt in the neck and shoulders may also affect the lower back and, conversely, hip and low back problems may be reflected in the upper body.

Getting the back balance right

As we have seen, our physical stresses and strains contribute to the pains we feel in our back, so the first thing we must do is think about the ways we use our bodies. Take time to look at yourself in a full-length mirror. What do you see? Draw an imaginary line down the centre of your body: is your body even and well balanced, or do the two halves look very different? Look at the spaces made between your arms and your body. How did you get this way?

Everyday imbalances

What are your habitual patterns of movement? Do you always cross your legs the same way, or stand with your weight on one leg? If you work at a word processing keyboard, is the chair the right height to enable you to look down at the screen, and if copytyping do you always turn your head to the same side? Do you carry bags or heavy objects always on one arm? Do you use a shoulder bag? These examples may be fairly obvious, but have you considered that the way you use your legs also affects your back and the balance of your body? If you run, walk a lot, and always wear heeled shoes, the backs of your legs may become tighter than the fronts and so exert an uneven pull on your pelvis.

Front versus back (*Right*) **Think about the balance between front and back musculature. Is your waist well defined? Turn sideways to the mirror and look at the balance between front and back. How much curve is there at the back of the waist? Does your bottom jut out? What about your tummy? If you detect imbalance here, follow the abdominal strengthening exercises as well as the back stretches (see pages 54 and 27).**

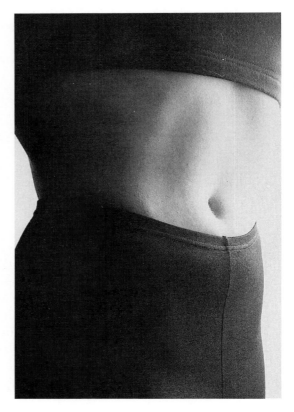

Warming up wisely and well

You may find some difficulty in actually reaching areas of back tension so, in order to get to all the parts of your back with your hands it will be necessary to warm up and stretch your shoulders. Begin with some shoulder shrugs, inhaling as you lift the shoulders towards your ears and exhaling as you let them drop. Follow with some shoulder circles, doing these slowly so that you get maximum movement. Inhale as your shoulders come forwards and exhale on the back and downwards movement. Now follow with this sequence of stretches:

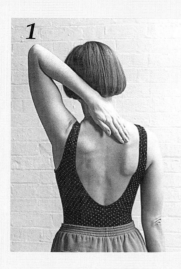

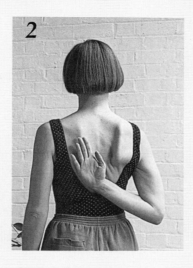

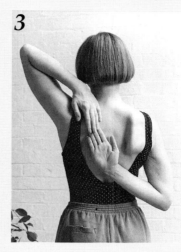

1 Raise your left arm and then bring your hand down behind your head to touch the right shoulder blade. Feel the stretch in the back of the upper arm.

2 Next, stretch your right arm to the side and twist it up behind your back to touch the left shoulder blade. Feel the stretch in the shoulder and perhaps in the wrist. Repeat these stretches on the other side.

3 Combine these stretches, aiming to touch your fingers behind your back. Do both sides. Often it is easier to one side than the other. To maintain full mobility of your shoulder joints, practise until the stretch becomes easy on both sides.

4 Clasp your hands lightly behind your back and, keeping your elbows bent, squeeze them towards each other. Feel an opening stretch in the chest and a tightening between the shoulder blades. Relax as the elbows move apart. Do this three or four times.

5 Draw your right arm across your body until you feel a stretch in the outer arm muscle and the back of the shoulder. Repeat on the other side.

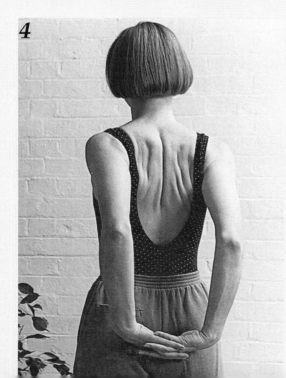

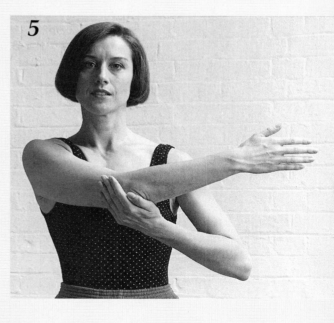

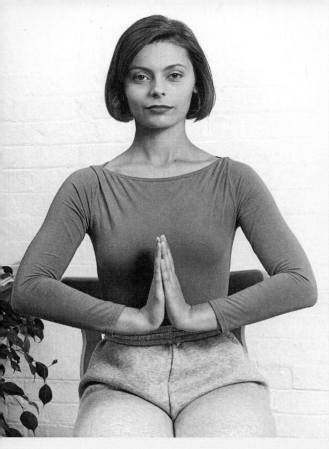

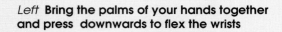

Left **Bring the palms of your hands together and press downwards to flex the wrists**

Below left **Then bring your elbows together**

Below **Keeping hands, forearms and elbows together, raise the hands up until you feel the stretch between your shoulder blades**

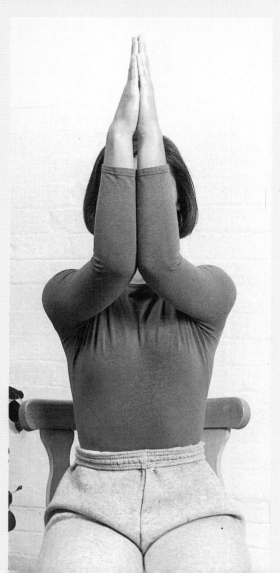

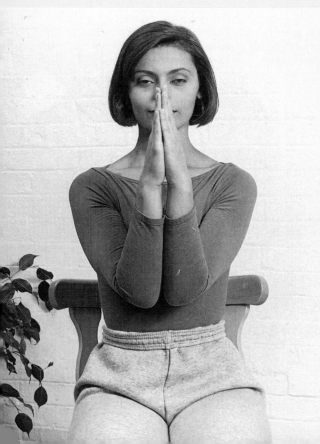

Getting down to your back

Simply slapping or tapping over the back can have a releasing and refreshing effect. In Oriental techniques, percussive movements are used to tone and invigorate the body and its internal organs by following the lines of energy flow known as *meridians.* To begin working on your back, try a form of this type of massage.

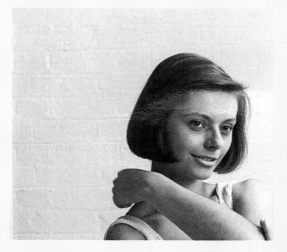

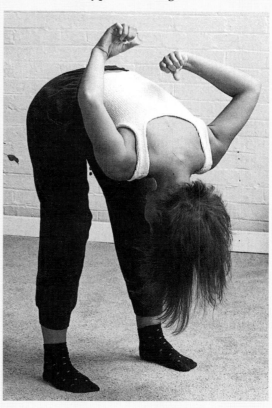

Above **Start by making light rapping movements with loosely-held fists on either side of your neck and onto your shoulders.**

Right **Now lean forward and, reaching up behind your back as high as possible, make percussive movements downwards along either side of the spine and onto each buttock, making the movements stronger over the larger muscles.**

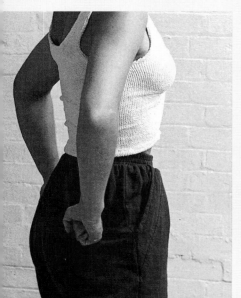

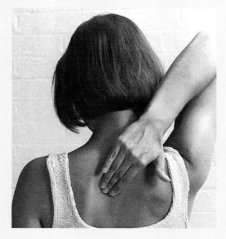

Far left **Loosen and relax these muscles by pushing your fists into the indentations at either side of the buttocks and rotating them.**

Left **Reach up behind your head to the muscles between your shoulder blades and perform circling movements (petrissage).**

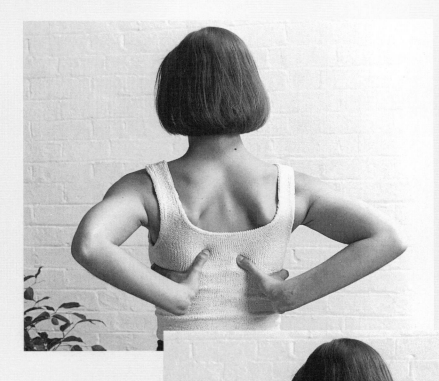

Left **Next use your thumbs and, reaching up behind your back as far as possible, start making thumb-circling movements into the muscles at either side of the spine. Make the pressure stronger and deeper if it feels good to do so.**

Right **Continue with your thumbs if this is comfortable, or change to finger circles when you reach waist level.**

When you reach the point where your spine joins your pelvis -- the sacrum -- change once again to thumb pressure. The sacrum feels like a flat triangle between your hip bones and has small holes, called foramen, which occur in pairs.

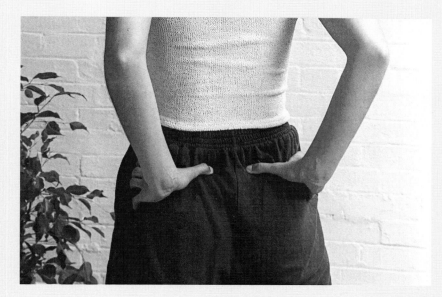

Left **Feel for these small holes with your thumbs and press into them. Pressure at these points is very beneficial to low back ache and also brings relief from period pains.**

Ball and wall techniques

Although all the forms of massage described above will help release tension in your back, the effort of reaching the appropriate spot may be just too much. In that case, you can use the 'ball-and-wall' technique. Take a bouncy rubber ball about the size of an orange, stand close to a wall and place the ball between your body and the wall.

Right **Lean against the ball to the required depth of pressure and rub yourself up and down like a bear against a tree.**

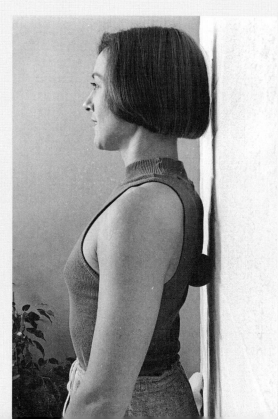

Rock and roll massage

As I have already pointed out, self-massage for the whole back is difficult to achieve -- so here's a method that gets to the parts that you can't reach. Make sure you have a firm, padded surface to cushion your spine. Lie down on your back, curl up and rock from side to side, then roll forwards and backwards. As the spine loosens up, the movement will become smoother and more controlled, and it is also very effective for conditioning the abdominal muscles!

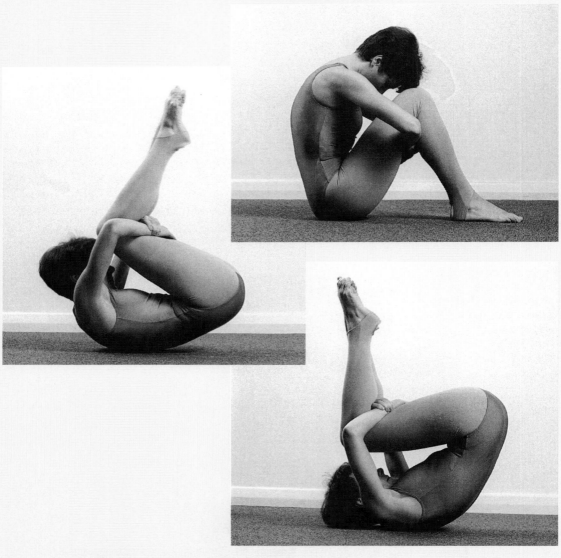

Once you have been through your back massage, you can then try out some or all of the following stretches to make your own routine:

Stretching it out

Right **Use pushing movements of your hands and arms to stretch out each side of your upper body. Standing comfortably erect, push upwards towards the ceiling with one hand as you push down towards the floor with the other. Feel the elongating stretch as your ribs lift up away from your hip bones. Repeat on the other side.**

Below **Stretch out your back using a chair for support. Rest your hands on the the back of the chair and, with your feet hip width apart, walk back until your back is flat like a table top. Try to keep your heels directly under your buttock bones. If the hamstring muscles in the backs of your legs are stiff, bend your knees a little to relax them. Feel the stretch in your back and maybe at the front of your shoulders.**

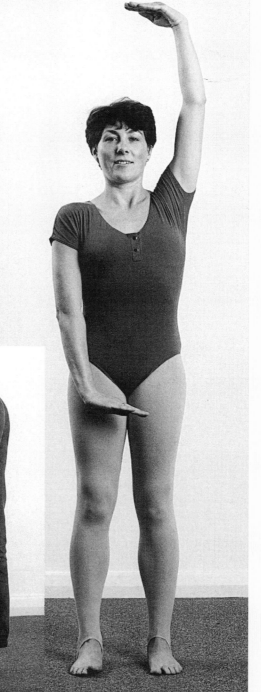

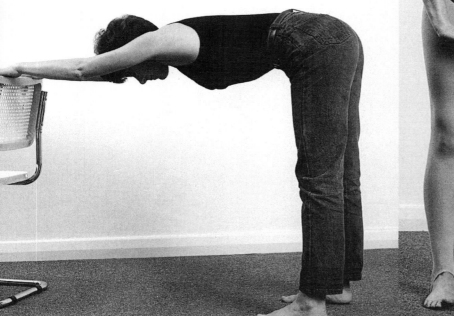

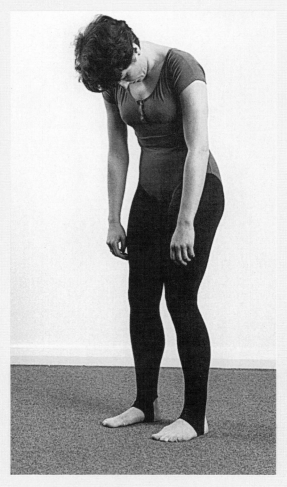

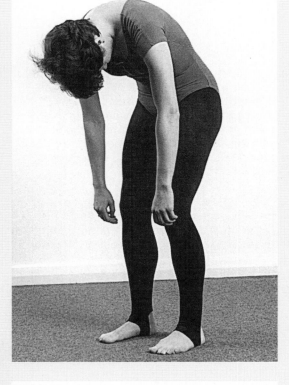

Use the "puppet stretch" to release and stretch the muscles of your hamstrings and back. Stand comfortably erect and imagine you are a stringed puppet. Gradually the strings become slack so that first your head, then shoulders and then upper back begin to droop forward. Continue this feeling to allow your upper body to roll right down to hang from the hips, bending your knees until your ribs touch your thighs. Allow your head to hang heavy towards the floor.

Relax more and more into this stretch and then *slowly* uncurl, bringing your head up last of all.

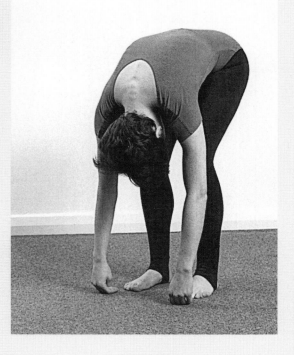

The next series of stretches are done on hands and knees. Make sure you are stretching on a padded surface so that you protect your knees. A yoga or exercise mat is ideal but a carpet is fine, or you could use a towel. Get onto all fours, having your knees under your hip joints and your hands directly under your shoulders. If you have difficulty in flexing your wrists, make fists and press the knuckles of your hands against the floor. Use this position as the start of each of the following stretches.

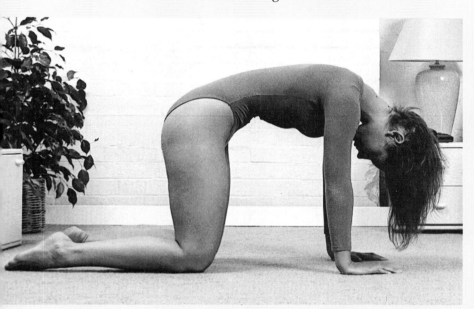

Left **Tuck your tail under and arch the middle of your back upwards, allowing your head to follow the curve of your spine and drop forwards.**

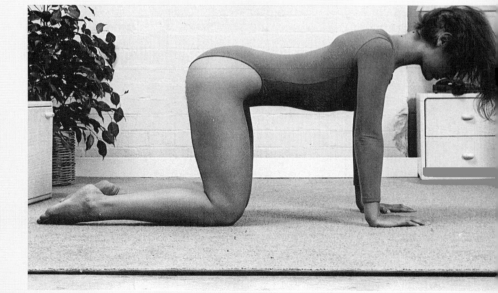

Right **Now begin to uncurl from your tail, allowing the middle of your back to sink down and your head to look upwards. Imagine a cat asking for cream! NB. If you have a lower back problem, bring your back to the "flat" position only.**

From the start position, it is possible to stretch the outer hips and buttock muscles simply by allowing the hips to roll towards the floor on either side of you whilst keeping the hands and arms stationary. Roll to the side and hold the stretch for about thirty seconds before returning to the starting position and rolling to the other side. If you repeat the stretch from side to side a few times, you will find that the movement becomes easier as the muscles relax and stretch and that your hips roll closer to the floor. From the same starting position move on to stretch the upper back with a twisting movement called "threading the needle".

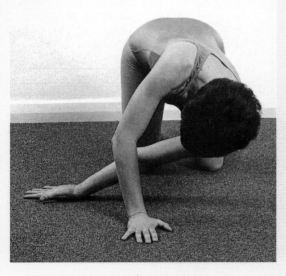
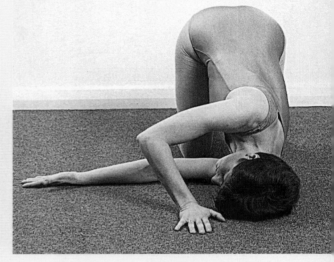

Above left & right **Slide your left arm through the space between your right hand and knee, continue the movement as far as you are comfortable. Feel the twist of the upper back and the stretch around the left shoulder blade. Repeat on the other side.**

Below **Finish this series of stretches by allowing your bottom to sink back onto your heels and your chest and arms to reach out forwards along your thighs and beyond.**

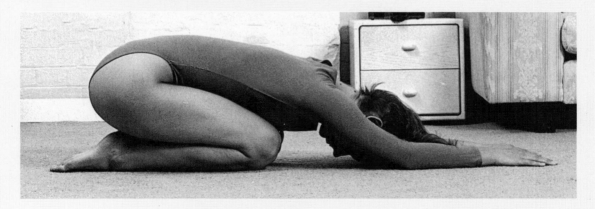

A very good way to stretch out the muscles of your back, particularly if you have back problems, is to do so from a supine position. Take time to settle into the start position, lying straight with knees bent to enable the small of your back to come in contact with the floor. Allow yourself to let go as much as possible so that the spinal vertebrae can sink down towards the floor. After you have finished the rolling up stretch, allow yourself to rest in this position for a few moments before continuing.

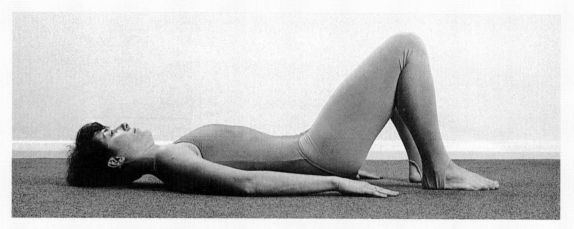

Above **Prepare with a few pelvic tilts, pressing the small of your back down into the floor and curling your pubic bone upwards. Feel as though you are about to lift your buttocks off the floor without actually doing so.**

Below **Now tilt your pelvis and slowly begin to peel your back off the floor, starting with your tailbone and gradually moving upwards vertebra by vertebra towards your upper back. Try to keep your head, neck and shoulders relaxed and to feel your lower back lengthening throughout. Return to the start position by reversing the process. Lengthen even more by imagining that your knees press forwards as you lower your back.**

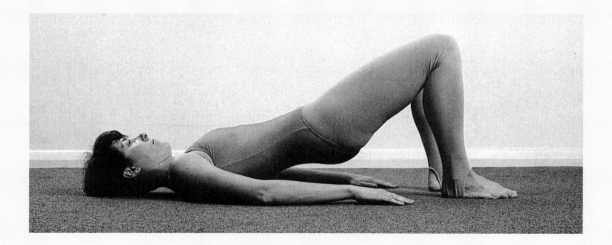

If you have sufficient space, finish your floor work with the "Space roll". I call it this because it feels weightless as if in space. Keep your body heavy and relaxed throughout the roll.

Right **Lying on your right side as shown, begin by lifting your left arm to make a half circle to the other side of your body.**

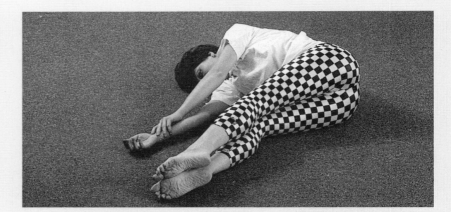

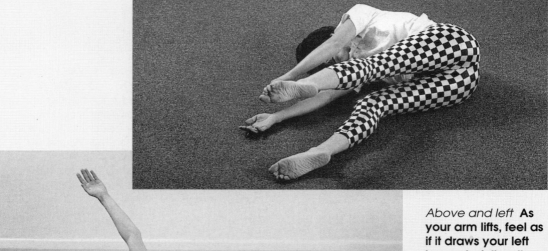

Above and left **As your arm lifts, feel as if it draws your left leg up to follow it. Continue making the half circle until your right leg feels obliged to follow.**

32

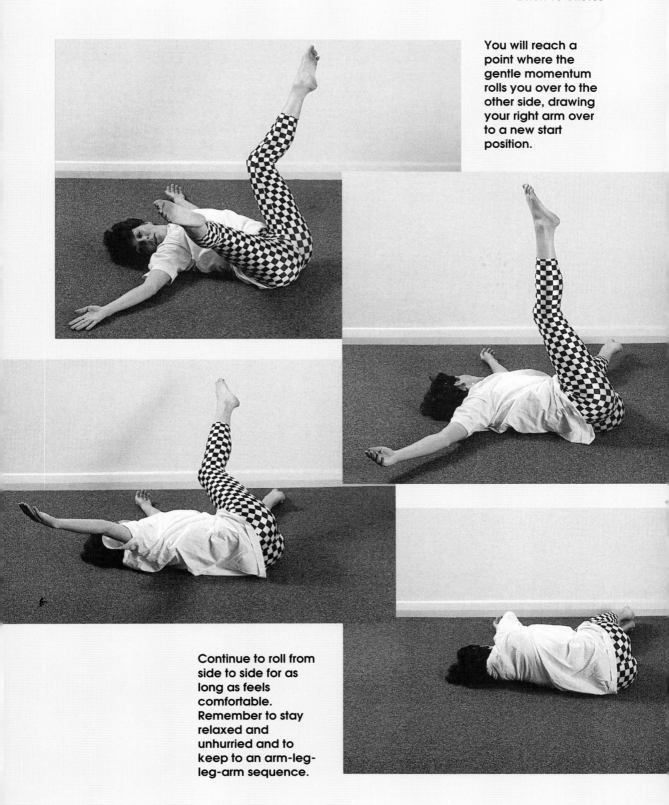

You will reach a point where the gentle momentum rolls you over to the other side, drawing your right arm over to a new start position.

Continue to roll from side to side for as long as feels comfortable. Remember to stay relaxed and unhurried and to keep to an arm-leg-leg-arm sequence.

Here's a routine which can even be used in the office. Sit comfortably erect on the front of your chair as shown below, and begin with a pelvic tilt, tucking your tailbone under and curling your pubic bone upwards. Press your waist back and draw in your abdominal muscles, and stretch forward with your clasped hands.

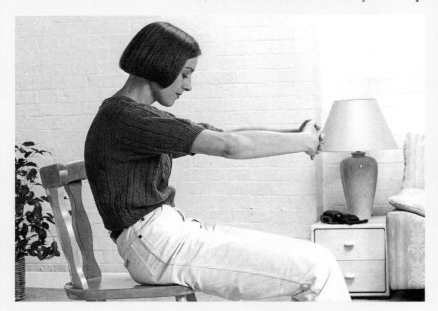

Left **During the pelvic tilt, feel a stretch in your back, especially between your shoulder-blades.**

Below **This is a seated version of the Puppet stretch (see p28). Beginning with your head, allow your body to roll down to hang from the hips. Feel the stretch in the whole spine and the back of your hips.**

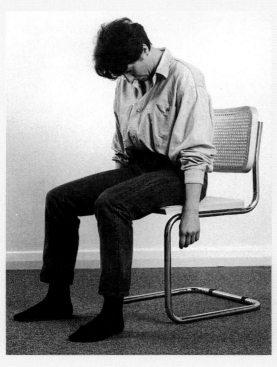

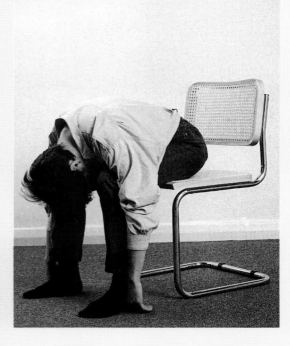

Right **Feel your hips and buttocks heavy as you lift upwards and bend towards the left side. Keep your back straight, abdominal muscles drawn in and bend directly to the side. Feel the stretch at the side of your waist. Repeat to the other side.**

Below left **For a stronger stretch, repeat with your right arm bent and your left hand braced on your hip. As you bend sideways, increase the stretch still further by pointing your right elbow up towards the ceiling. Repeat to the other side.**

Below right **Finally, lift upwards as before and, keeping the feeling of lift, turn so that your shoulders and upper back face to the right. Your arms may be used to assist the stretch as shown. Again, repeat the stretch to the other side.**

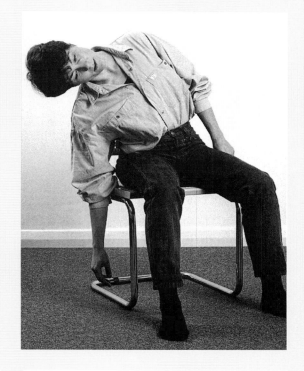

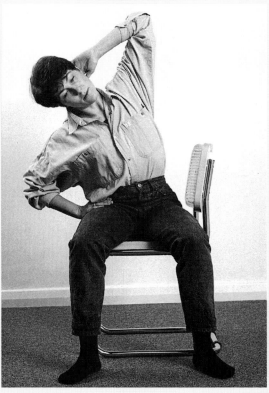

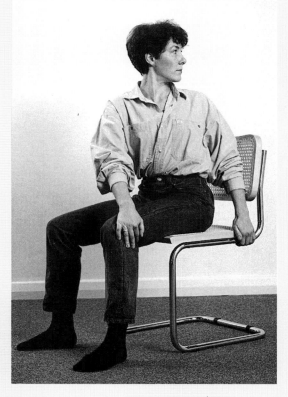

The power of effective visualisation

Bodywork methods such as Alexander and Feldenkrais techniques, which work on posture and the natural balance of the body, use visualisation techniques. Indeed, it has been proven that relaxing body and mind and imagining certain feelings or visualising changes within the body can actually alter structure -- given time. Remember how you assessed yourself standing before a full-length mirror? What changes would you like to make -- and be realistic! When you can make a space of about 15 minutes for yourself, try the following:

Lie on your back with knees bent so that your feet rest on the floor and the hollow at the back of your waist disappears. If you have a big hollow, you may need to place a cushion under your pelvis, or raise your legs so that they rest on a chair, knees bent at right angles so that the spine touches the floor. If your chin points upwards towards the ceiling you may need to place a folded towel or one or two paperback books under your head so that the back of your neck is elongated.

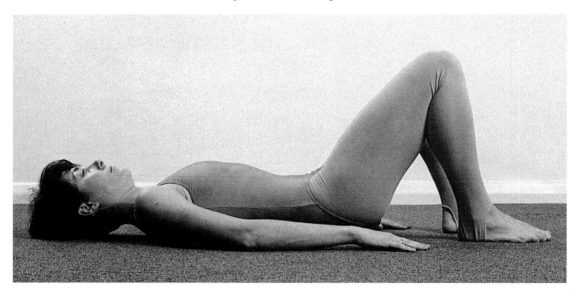

Towards total relaxation

Be aware of your breathing and allow it to slow down. Placing your hands on your lower ribs, focus your attention there and see if you can allow the breath to expand the ribs sideways as you inhale, letting them move inwards with the exhalation. Bring your hands down to rest on your tummy and allow your attention and breath to focus there. Allow any minor irritations and twitches to happen and then let them subside until you feel relaxed, your breath is slow and easy, and all the little bones of your spine feel as if they are sinking towards the floor.

Verbalise what you want

Now begin to visualise or imagine your supple body and the ease with which it moves. If you have difficulty in imagining this, try saying to yourself the improvements you would like to make. For instance you may say "my shoulders are moving up and back so that my chest is open and free. The muscles of my back are releasing and softening", or something along these lines. You may find that soft music aids this process, or you may wish to make a tape repeating out loud to yourself the improvements that you most want.

Ending the session

Once you have finished your period of relaxation and visualisation, allow yourself time to come back to your normal breathing pattern, take a long stretch and roll onto your side before sitting and standing up so that you don't come to earth with a jolt. Whenever you can remember during the day, remind yourself of your long, supple back — and walk and sit tall.

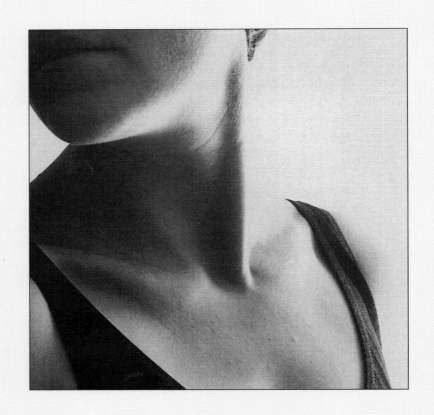

3
Pain in the Neck

Are all your anxieties carried as a burden on your shoulders? Massaging and stretching your neck will help you lighten the load.

Physical and emotional anatomy

The neck is the only highway between the organising centre of the brain and the rest of the body. All traffic (the air we breathe, nerve impulses, blood, lymph etc) passes through this narrow route; because of this, it easily becomes congested. Obstructions occur from physical causes, such as carrying a heavy bag, a briefcase or a small child, but they can also have emotional causes. Coping with the sort of person we call "a pain in the neck", biting back angry responses or holding back tears and fears will all cause muscle contraction and tension and changes in our breathing. We may unconsciously hold our breath and thus contribute even more stress to the body.

Building up tension

How is it that tension can creep up on us almost unawares until it results in pain? The problem is that the brain registers the position of our joints but not the tension in our muscles. Tension may thus become chronic, interfering with the circulation of blood and lymph, restricting joint mobility and pulling the body out of alignment; all this can happen before the brain recognises the situation and we feel warning signals of pain in the areas affected.

What can we do about this? By using a combination of self-massage, stretch, breathing and visualisation, we can not only alleviate the discomfort of muscular tension but also reach a deeper level of body-mind awareness, contributing to the maintenance of holistic health and well being.

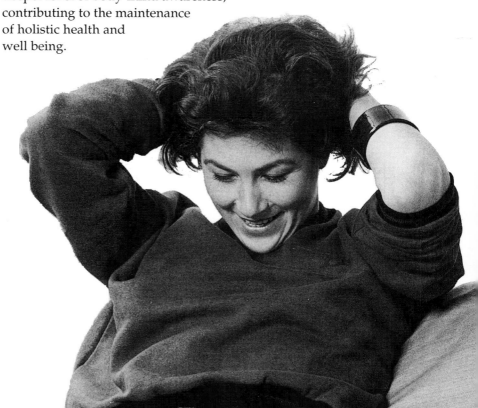

**Stretch, breathe
and smile.
How does it feel --
better ?**

Breathing and tension release -- the 'triangle' visualisation

In tense and stressful situations we may find our heart rate and breathing becoming faster, or we may 'freeze' and hold our breath. Try this experiment: inhale and hold the breath. Notice how the neck, shoulders and facial muscles become fixed and stiff. Now exhale through the mouth with a sigh and notice how these muscles soften. Inhale again and, exhaling on a sigh, visualise a triangle which encloses your head and shoulders. Imagine the top of your head moving upwards to the apex while the shoulders move downwards to the angles at the base. Notice how the neck feels. Because the muscles of the neck and shoulders have this close relationship with the way you breathe, take a moment to register how your breath feels before you perform your self-massage, and again afterwards.

Tension release through massage

All the muscles which attach the head to the upper body pass through the neck and then fan outwards onto the back and shoulders. For this reason, the neck cannot be dealt with in isolation, so before attempting any massage, warm up the shoulders with a few shrugs and circles. These moves can be made whilst wearing clothing and some of them are easier without using oil. Follow the stroke sequence of stroking, kneading and/or tapotement and petrissage.

Making a start

Begin by stroking down the side of your neck and out across the shoulder.

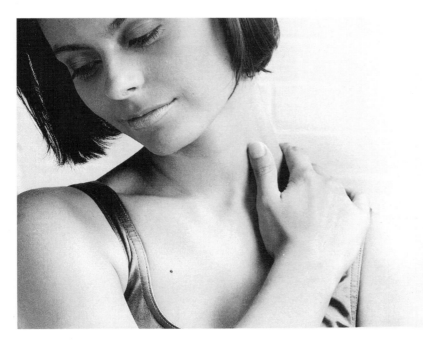

Left **Stroke down the side of your neck and shoulders. Use alternate hands and sides to produce a gentle rhythm. Keep your hands and fingers relaxed and moulded to the body contours.**

Right **Squeeze and knead into the muscle at the top of your left shoulder, then repeat on the other side.**

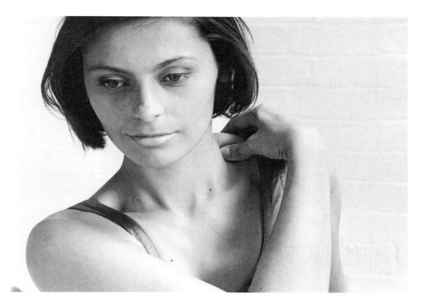

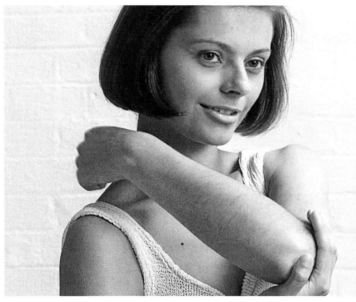

Left **If it feels very tense, add some slapping or tapping movements as if you were giving yourself a pat on the back.**

Going deeper

Knead again and begin to feel deeper for the little knots of tautness, those areas which are painful to the touch and are the focus of much tension, especially after a hard day's work.

Next, locate the largest of these knots and, holding it in thumb and fingers, begin to circle the shoulder backwards and forwards. As you do so, you allow the movement of the shoulder to create its own massage and you will feel the muscle stretching and relaxing.

Having dealt with the tension in the muscle at the top of the shoulder, relax the massaging hand and allow the fingers to creep down the back and onto the shoulder blade.

Right **With your fingers, explore the triangular shape of the shoulder-blade and make petrissage movements into any areas of tenderness. These areas may be particularly obvious near the ridge of the shoulder blade. Repeat this sequence for the other shoulder.**

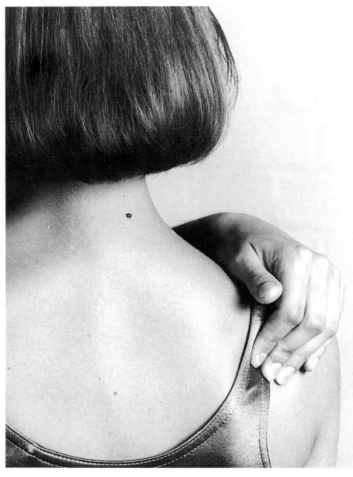

Breathing easy

Once you have completed the massage, check how your breath feels. Is it free and effortless? As you breathe, are you aware of the spaces within the head, the mouth, throat and chest? If the breath still feels restricted, take a cupped hand and make percussive tapping movements over the whole area of the lungs. You may be surprised at the area they cover as you tap over the top of the shoulders (deep 'salt cellars' indicate that this part of the lung does not get used in breathing), across the chest, along the lower ribs and at the side of the body above the waist.

Now check your breathing again -- has it become easier? Continue with the 'anywhere' stretch routine given on page 44.

Right **Place the fingertips of both hands on either side of the neck and make little petrissage movements into the muscles.**

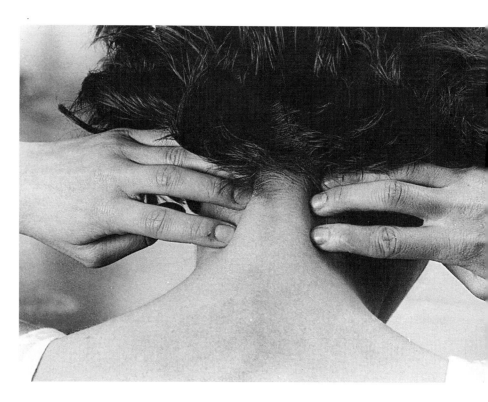

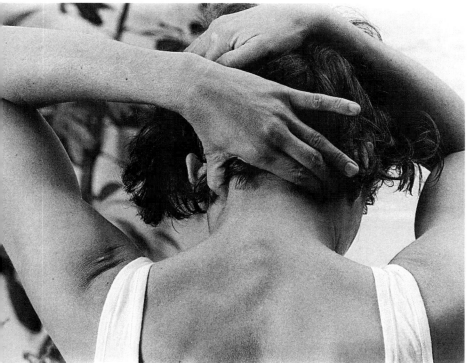

Left **Lift and gently pull the scruff of the neck a few times and then, taking hold of the scruff, make small nodding movements, followed by turns from side to side as if saying 'no'. Once again the movements create the deeper massage.**

To finish, soothe the muscles with long stroking effleurage movements. You can use the ball-and-wall massage (see page 25) for the back of the neck and shoulders.

The 'anywhere' stretch routine

This stretch routine can be performed in almost any situation -- at home, in the office, travelling or whenever you feel tension creeping up into your neck and shoulders. Sit comfortably erect with your weight taken on your sitting bones, feet flat on the floor with your knees in line with your hips and your feet in line with and slightly forward of your knees.

Start with a few deep breaths, some shoulder shrugs and the triangle visualisation (see page 40). Keep the feeling of length through the neck during the following stretches, which use the weight of the head and gravity to release tense muscles.

Left **Turn your head slowly from side to side. Note the range of movement and any 'noises' you hear in your head!**

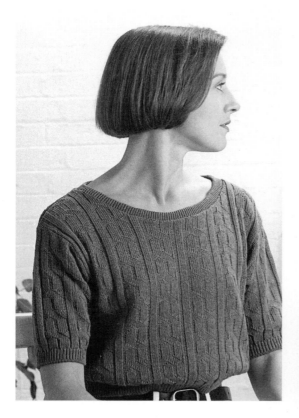

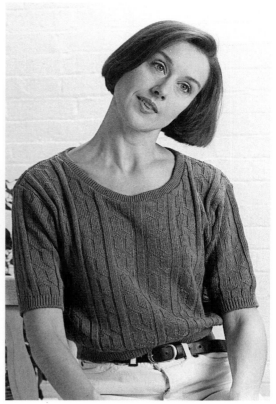

Right **Keep your chin tucked in, exhale and allow the left ear to move towards the left shoulder. Hold this position, allowing the outbreath to aid further release of the muscles. Focus attention on the side of the neck and imagine you can breathe the tension out through that part.**

When the stretch feels complete, inhale and as you exhale bring the head to an upright position. Repeat the stretch on the right side.

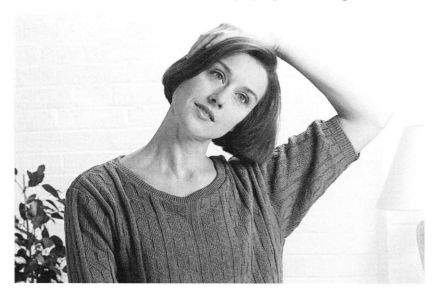

To increase the stretch, bring your left hand to rest on the side of your head, fingertips towards your ear. Stay relaxed and allow the weight of your hand and arm to gradually stretch further. Remember not to pull with your hand. Repeat on the other side.

Still keeping the neck long, allow your chin to move towards your chest, breathing out as you do so. Hold the position for a while and when the stretch feels complete, inhale and as you exhale bring your head upright.

Repeat the movement, visualising a long, graceful neck such as that of a swan or a racehorse, and feel the movement begin between your shoulder-blades. Bring your head to an upright position as before.

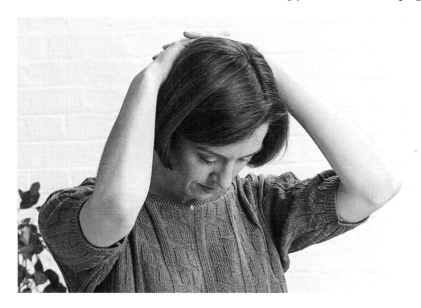

To stretch further, clasp your hands lightly and place them on the back of your head. Then repeat the stretch movement and, without pulling on the head, bring your elbows towards your face. Keep your hands and arms relaxed throughout.

The forward tilt of the head can also be done on the diagonal. Turn your head a quarter turn to the right and lower your chin onto your chest. Hold this position and breathe as before, then return your head to upright and face front. Repeat to the other side.

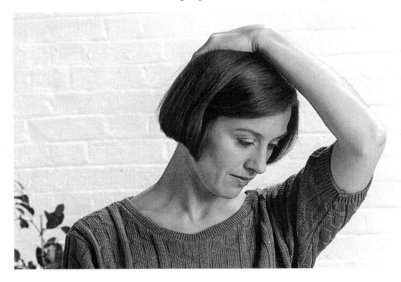

To stretch further, fold your arm across your head and bring your chin towards your chest.

Before the next stretch, loosen the area between your shoulder-blades as described in the warming-up routine on page 21.

From your upright sitting posture, breathe out and allow your pelvis to tilt so that your tail bone curls underneath and your pubic bone curls upwards. Your back should feel rounded and your stomach muscles should feel pulled in. Inhale as you return to the upright position.

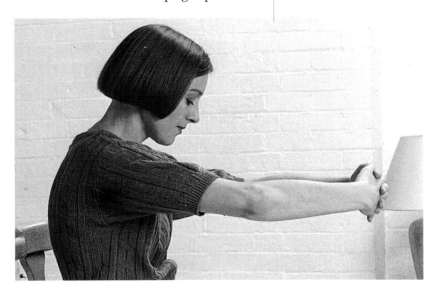

Tilt your pelvis and push forward with your clasped hands until you feel a stretch between your shoulder blades.

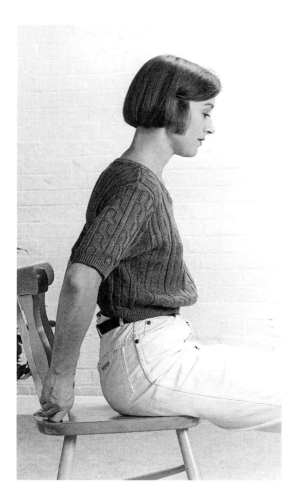

Left **Sitting in an upright posture as before, place your hands at the back of your chair for support. Stretch your back upwards, lift your breastbone up towards the ceiling and tilt your head to look upwards. Remember to keep your neck lengthened so that you don't scrunch the neck bones.**

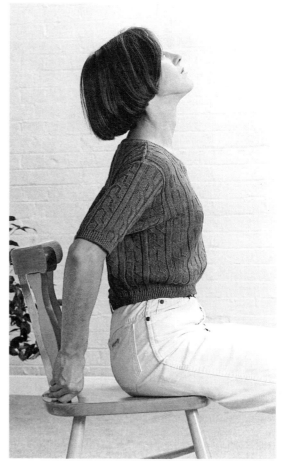

Right **Still looking upwards, take an imaginary bite out of the ceiling, or repeat a resonating "Umm" a few times, feeling a stretch at the front of the throat. Return to the upright on an inbreath.**

Lastly, sit comfortably erect and slowly turn your head from side to side. Note the ease and quality of the movement. Close your eyes and for a few moments imagine what it would be like if you had no bones in your neck, and your head was balanced on a piece of rubber tubing. When you open your eyes again, slowly turn your head again and notice any changes.

The above sequence of stretches form a routine which can be done anywhere, but when you have time and space, you can add some floorwork to this routine.

A really effective way of releasing tension in the neck and shoulder area is to use the 'Rainbow stretch'. I call it this because you draw a rainbow shape around your head as you stretch.

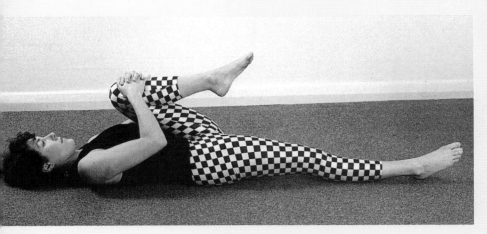

1 Start by lying supine and allow your back to elongate and sink into the floor. Draw your left knee up towards your chest.

2 and 3 Stretch your left arm to your side and carefully draw your left knee across your body towards the floor as you turn your head to the left.

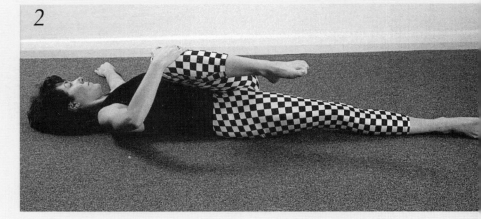

2

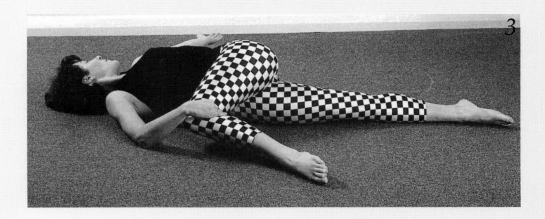

3

4 and 5 Bring your left hand down to touch your back, then begin to draw the rainbow around your head, keeping the back of your hand on the floor.

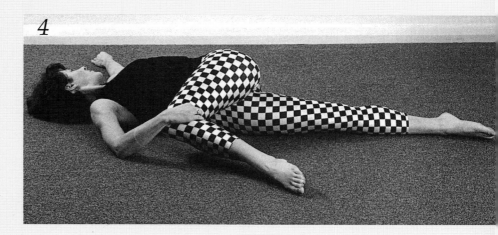

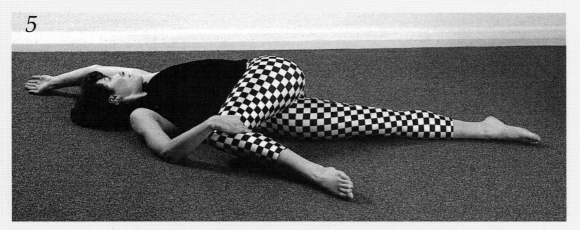

6 Allow your head to follow the movement and finish looking to the right with your left hand touching your left knee. Reverse the process to draw your hand back in an arc over your head until it touches your back again. Repeat the whole stretch and then repeat on the other side.

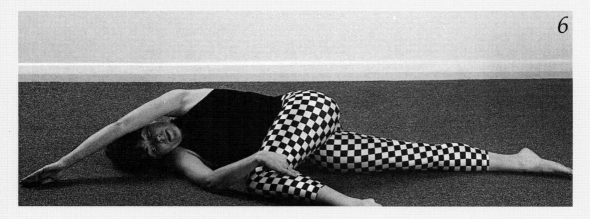

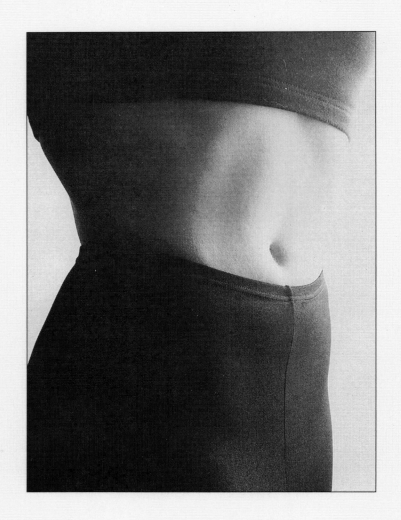

4

Gut reaction

*So much tension manifests in the pit of the stomach
that it's worth while learning how to get rid of it!*

Getting to the centre of things

Most of our physical tensions are felt in the back of the body. Our emotional ones, however, are felt in the front, in the area beneath the ribs known as the solar plexus.

When dealing with the centre of the body, it is necessary to employ different tactics from those we have already described, since there are other forces at play than simple muscular over-use and over-contraction. These forces are far less tangible and, although self-massage and stretching are undoubtedly helpful, we need to use other methods as well.

Everyone nevertheless seems to understand what we mean when we use a phrase such as "My gut reaction tells me that this would not be a good move." When we speak of a 'gut reaction', we generally mean some sort of instinctive feeling that seems to come from the centre of our being. Yet because it has to do with feelings and emotion and appears to have little connection with logic, such a reaction is difficult to describe or explain.

Strategies for stress

The solar plexus, commonly known as the pit of the stomach, may be seen as an important switchboard signalling the primitive reactions to stress -- the 'flight or fight' response -- and also the functioning of the organs of the abdominal area, such as the movement of food through the digestive tract, the filtering and excretory actions of the kidneys and the removal of toxins by the liver. Under stress, these functions may shut down or over-react. If we find it difficult to relax, digestive problems, including ulcers, may result. Thus there is a strong link between the emotional reaction and the physical response.

The strategies for dealing with both emotional and physical stress involve awareness and relaxation techniques which bring harmony to mind and body. Let's consider these first before moving to the touch techniques. The quickest way to achieve this harmony is through the breathing, since the brain produces powerful mood regulators according to the amount of oxygen and carbon dioxide in the blood.

The middle ground: looking and feeling good

The solar plexus lies close to the diaphragm -- the muscle responsible for our breathing. Since this muscle is attached to the spine, it affects both breathing and posture and thus our ability to relax effectively. One of the first noticeable effects of stress is a change in the way we breathe. Our breath becomes faster and mainly in the chest. This is a natural response, and only becomes a problem when stress continues over a long period and we fail to return to a deeper breathing pattern. We recognise the value of deeper breathing in such commands as "Take a deep breath and count to ten" before reacting to an emotional situation. A deep breath is also advocated to help counteract the nervousness we feel prior to events such as public speaking or interviews.

Breathing

Sometimes just by placing the flat of your hand over your solar plexus area you can bring awareness to that part and deeper breathing will follow. If this strategy does not work, try the following:

Take a wide tie belt and place it around your body at the level of your lower ribs. Cross the ends of the belt but do not tie it.

Exhale completely while drawing the ends of the belt apart so that you feel your ribs move inwards.

Inhale again, allowing the breathing movement to push against the belt as the ribs lift up and out and the ends of the belt move closer once more.

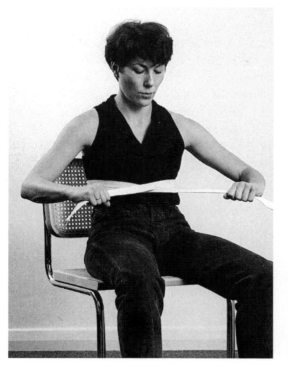
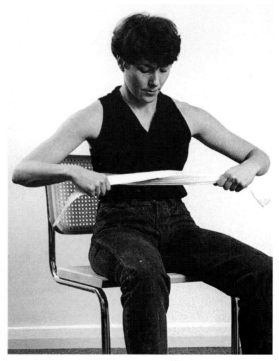

Repeat until your breathing feels full and natural. If it remains restricted, try the cupped hand percussion over the lung area described on page 42.

Posture

Now that you are breathing from the diaphragm, check your posture. Good posture makes for good breathing and also has an effect on our view of ourselves, our self-esteem and our emotional welfare: if we believe that we look good, we feel good. So:

Stand sideways before a mirror; with feet hip-width apart and knees relaxed, notice your body alignment, particularly in the pelvis area.

Place your hands one in front and one behind your body with fingers pointing downwards, and tilt your pelvis back and forth. Is this movement easy, or does it feel stiff?

Continue the pelvic tilting movements and note how your back shortens and arches and your stomach protrudes when the tail sticks out, and how your stomach flattens and your back lengthens when the tail is tucked under.

Now find the point where your pelvis feels balanced and your tail bone is centred, neither tucked under nor tilted back.

Visualisation exercises

Imagine that your body is in segments like building blocks and line up the box of your ribs over your pelvis. Now imagine lengthening your back to create more space at your waist and, still lengthening upwards, balance your head at the top. This may feel a little strange at first: you may feel as if you are leaning forwards, but if you look in the mirror, you should see an improvement in your stance. In order to maintain this posture as you move through your daily life, try these visualisation exercises: you may find one or all of them helpful.

1) To maintain the position of your pelvis, imagine that you have a spotlight on the end of your tail bone and that your feet are always in this light. If you allow your tail to stick out, the light will fall behind you: if you tuck under too much, the light will fall in front.

2) To maintain a feeling of length in your back, imagine yourself as the gooey, creamy filling between two layers of cake. Turn the cake on end and imagine the piece of cake at your back sliding downwards over the filling.

3) To maintain the balance of your head, imagine that you have two faces, one at the front and one at the back. Keep both sets of eyes and their sightlines level whatever direction you turn.

Strengthening the centre

Turn sideways to your mirror once more and take a critical look at the middle of your body and the balance between the muscles of your back and those of your abdomen. For most people, the back muscles are the stronger ones and the abdomen may protrude. If this is the case for you, strengthen the abdominal muscles with the exercises outlined below.

For all these exercises, make sure that the small of your back is pressed into the floor and that you breathe out as you contract the muscles. Do not pull on your head as you curl up, keep the movement smooth. Make each movement several times and build up the repetitions as your muscles get stronger.

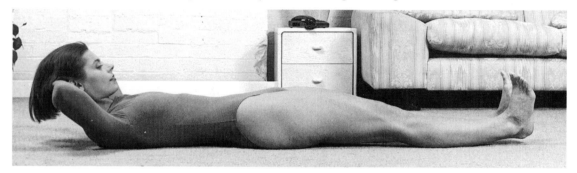

Above **Start lying supine and relaxed, head resting in your hands. As you breathe out, flatten your back into the floor, flex your ankles and lift your head to look at your toes.** **Breathe in as you relax. Repeat at least eight times.**

Right **With knees bent, breathe out and lift your head and shoulders off the floor. Breathe in as you relax. Repeat eight times as before.**

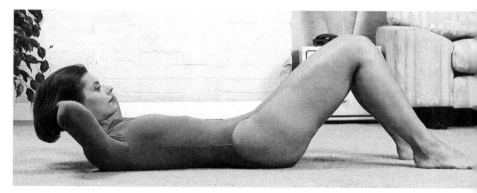

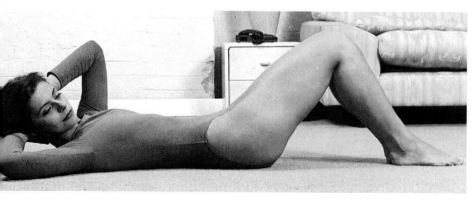

Left **As you breathe out, lift and turn diagonally to point your left elbow towards your right knee. Breathe in to relax and repeat to the other side. Do both sides at least eight times.**

Right **Lie on your side as shown, extending your body in a straight line. If you have a deep curve at the back of your waist, bring your legs forward a little so that your back is straight.**

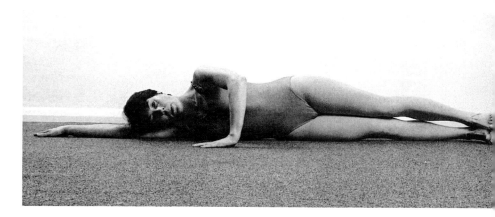

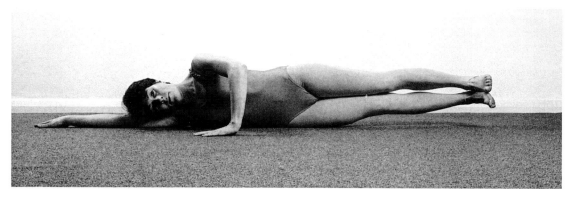

Above **Breathe out and, drawing in your abdominal muscles, lift both legs a little off the floor. Breathe in and relax to the start position.**

Since we have already considered the pelvis, we should think a little about the muscles which make up the floor of the pelvis and literally hold everything up. If these muscles are not in good shape, then our abdominal organs are not held in their best position and tend to sag downwards. In women the consequences may be a prolapsed womb with pressure upon the bladder, which may possibly require surgery. It therefore makes sense to do a few exercises to prevent this happening. Usually these exercises are taught to women in their pre- and post-natal periods, but they are not for women only -- men, too, can benefit.

The muscles in the pelvic floor are strengthened in the same way as other muscles, by contracting them. Many people, however, find them difficult to locate, and it may be easier to start with the anal sphincter, the muscle which closes the back passage. Contract this muscle, feel the squeeze and bring the squeezing sensation forward towards the pubic bone at the front of the pelvis. The feeling should be one of lifting upwards inside the body and though it may feel weak at first, like any other muscle it responds to challenge by growing stronger.

Massage techniques for the abdomen

Now we are ready to move on to the touch techniques, the stretches, and some ways of dealing with stress using aromatherapy.

Self-massage for the abdominal area is easy compared with reaching some parts of the back, and employs less strokes. You can perform this massage directly over clothing, or using oil or lotion directly on the skin, or using soap or shower gel while you are bathing. Make each of the movements several times.

Use thumb pressures over the ball of your foot or palm of your hand to massage the reflexes of the abdominal area (see reflexology chart, p.67). Massage particularly well into the area illustrated, as this is the solar plexus reflex and is a good tension relief point.

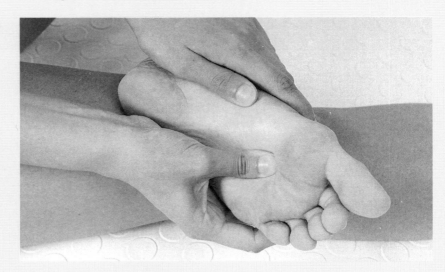

For direct massage, start with both hands on the chest with the heels of the hands pointing towards your armpits. Sweep your hands out and down the sides of your body to your hips, keeping your hands relaxed and moulded to the contours of your body.

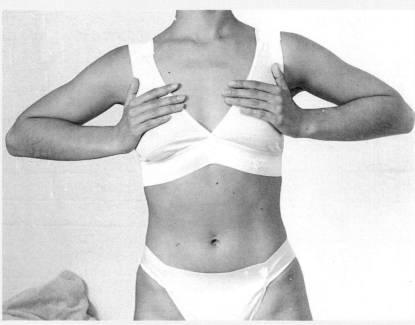

Bring your hands inwards to the centre and, placing one hand over the other with fingers pointing downwards, draw them up the mid-line of your body until they reach the starting point again. Put the emphasis of your stroke on the upward movement.

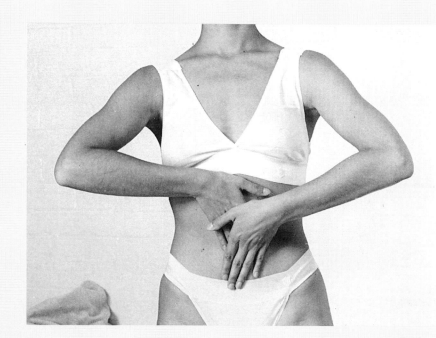

Now place your hands one above the other and circle around the abdomen in a clockwise direction, feeling into the contours of the hip bones and the rib cage.

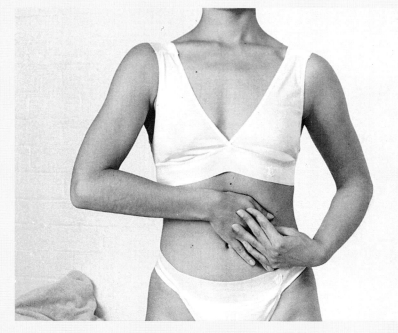

Finally, with hands held one over the other, massage over the navel with a push-and-pull action to give a rocking sensation. Push inwards and slightly upwards with the heel of the leading hand, then release pressure before pulling inwards and upwards with the fingers.

Stretching out your stress

In order to stretch the abdomen, it is necessary to flex the back muscles. As you do so, take care of your back by imagining it lengthening all the time so that your vertebrae don't scrunch into each other at the back of your waist.

Use the stretches described in chapter 2 and add floor work as follows.

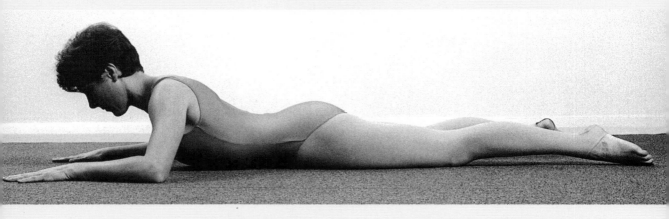

Above **Lying prone with forearms resting on the floor, breathe in and imagine yourself lengthening from the crown of your head. Raise your upper body as far as your lower ribs, breathing out as you slowly lower. If your back feels comfortable, proceed to the next stretch.**

Below **Repeat the stretch, this time lifting as far as your hips and extending your arms, but do not lift your hip bones off the floor. Feel the stretch at the front of your body.**

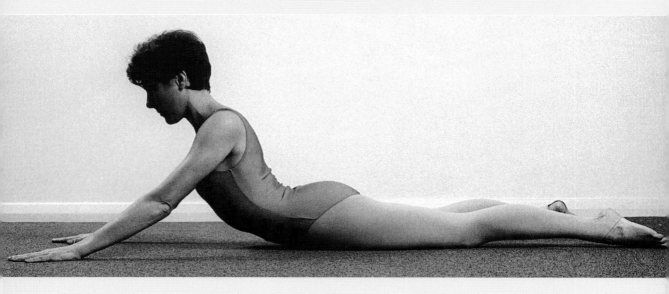

After flexing your back muscles, lengthen them again in a counter-stretch. The stretch illustrated is known as 'the pose of a child' in yoga. However, if you are not comfortable sitting back on your heels, lie on your back and hug your knees to your chest so that you feel your lower back stretch out.

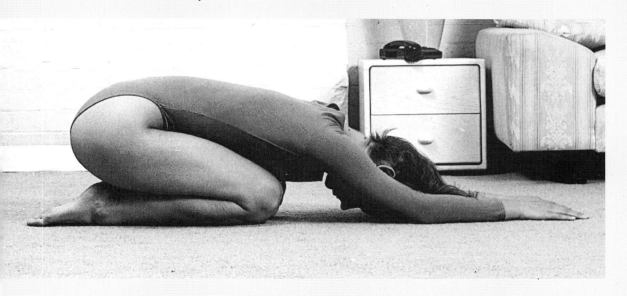

Above **Sit back on your heels and slide your arms forward until your ribs touch your thighs. Rest and breathe, imagining yourself reaching further forwards on each outbreath.**

Below **When your back has extended as far as possible, allow your arms to come back to your sides. Take several good breaths, aiming to feel the expansion in your back every time you breathe inwards.**

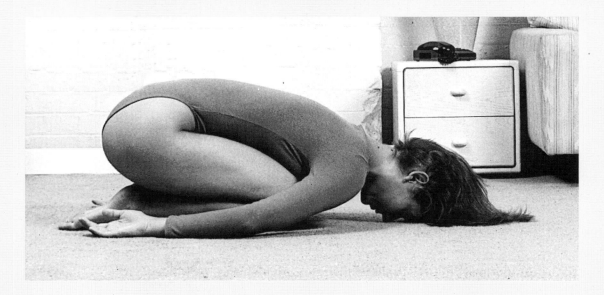

Finding a breathing space

The knot of anxiety felt in the pit of the stomach is best released by taking the time to relax, breathe and visualise. When you have little time to spare, follow the age-old advice and simply take two or three really deep breaths, concentrating fully on the process. If you feel fraught and hemmed in by people and events, use the bubble visualisation: as you breathe out, imagine blowing out a lovely iridescent bubble that completely surrounds you and separates you from everything round you. Make the bubble as large or as small as you feel necessary: when particularly hemmed in, I even imagine spikes on the outside of mine!

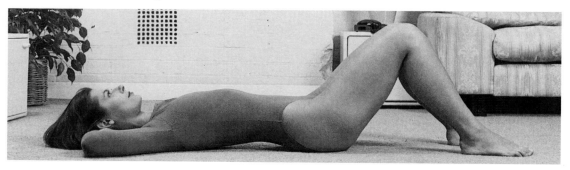

When you have time and space to lie down for ten minutes or more, try the following exercise known as the 'pelvic clock', which comes from the Feldenkrais method.

Lie supine as shown. Allow yourself time to breathe slowly and deeply and let your back settle well into the floor. When you are ready, imagine a clock face on your pelvis. Imagine twelve o'clock at the back of your waist, six o'clock at your tail bone, three o'clock at your left hip and nine o'clock at your right hip. Now press your back downwards at twelve and then slowly transfer the pressure to six o'clock, then back to twelve. This is a familiar movement for most people, so take time to *really* feel the slow change of pressure from one point to the next. Do the same for pressure between three and nine o'clock, again concentrating on the feeling as you move between the points.

Once these two basic movements are established and comfortable, try more difficult combinations. For example, press at one o'clock and transfer to seven o'clock several times. As you move across the clockface with varying combinations, you will find that some movements are relatively easy while others feel very restricted. Check these feelings by pressures going all the way round the clock, both clockwise and anti-clockwise. See if you can discover ways to relax and make the movements smoother and easier.

When you wish to finish the exercise, return to the starting position and rest for the space of several deep breaths so that your muscles are able to relax completely.

Use aromatherapy to banish tension

Because of its strong emotional factor, tension caused by stress is particularly helped with the use of aromatherapy. The essential oils may be diluted and applied to the skin, or they may be added to a relaxing bath. In either case you will benefit both from the effects of the aroma and the penetration of therapeutic substances into the bloodstream. The list of symptoms and appropriate oils which follows is meant as a guide and may be supplemented by experimenting to find the oils which suit you best and which you enjoy the most.

RECOMMENDED ESSENTIAL OILS

Symptom	Type of oil		
	Floral	Herbal	Exotic
Anti-depressant	Lavender Geranium	Clary Sage Melissa Jasmine	Sandalwood Ylang ylang Patchouli
	A combination of Clary Sage and Ylang ylang is particularly pleasing and helpful as an anti-depressant.		
Against anxiety	Rose Jasmine Neroli	Camomile Clary Sage Marjoram	
	All of these are costly -- so do not use them if your anxieties are to do with money!	*Any of the sedative and anti-depressant oils are also effective.*	
Sleep problems	Lavender	Marjoram	
Headache	Lavender	Peppermint	
	Applied neat over the temples	*Applied together with lavender, especially if the headache has a digestive origin*	
*Raised blood pressure	Lavender	Marjoram	Ylang ylang
	* Essential oils are useful in this situation, but thought needs to be given to general lifestyle and diet. Self-treatment is not a substitute for medical care.		

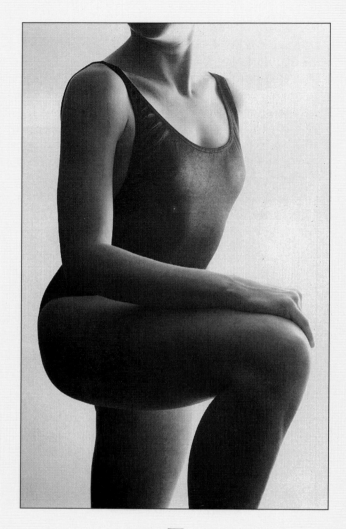

5
Out on a limb

*'Without the action of our arms and legs,
our powers are nothing.'*

Keeping our extremities in good shape

For me, being "out on a limb" evokes images of adventure, heroes and heroines hanging desperately to the branch of a tree to escape the gaping abyss or the jaws of a tiger. It means being at the extremities of experience, and such extremities tend to become pushed to the back of our minds. In the case of our own limbs, the extremities tend to be overlooked because of their very basic function in our daily lives.

Therapies such as reflexology which deal with the body's energy systems identify lines of energy (called meridians) which run through the body and can be affected and revitalised by massage of the hands and feet and their reflex points. To obtain the full therapeutic effect of reflexology -- also known as zone therapy -- you should seek out a qualified practitioner. In terms of self-help, however, there are a number of simple techniques which you can use at home and even in public.

Putting your best foot forward

Our feet play an important part in our posture and the whole way we present ourselves. Remember the times you have walked too far in new shoes? The visible signs of discomfort in your posture and expression must have been plain for all to see, and the eventual relief of kicking off those shoes and letting your feet expand was sheer bliss.

How our feet affect our posture

Perfect alignment of our body structure should be effortless, the bones aligned so that all is supported and balanced on the legs and feet. Our feet are wonderfully complex in their design, with arches to support and cushioning pads to take our weight. When the arches drop, or the feet roll inwards, our whole physical structure is thrown off balance: the knees tend to roll inwards, causing changes in the alignment of the hips; the lower back tends to arch, the bottom to push back while the stomach sags forward. If our stance is not corrected, the body seeks to return to a better position by giving more muscle to the thighs, and 'jodhpur thighs' may develop. Thus, working on the feet rather than following a tough exercise workout may be the cure for large thighs.

The following sequence of simple movements helps to make the feet supple and strong and will also help to correct a tendency to dropped arches. You may find it difficult to balance at first, so use the back of a chair for support.

Lifting your arches and strengthening your feet

Start by standing comfortably erect, pelvis centred and your knees relaxed.

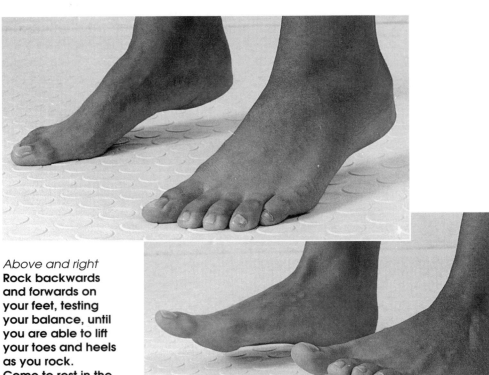

Above and right
**Rock backwards and forwards on your feet, testing your balance, until you are able to lift your toes and heels as you rock.
Come to rest in the centre, so that you are neither in front of nor behind your point of balance.**

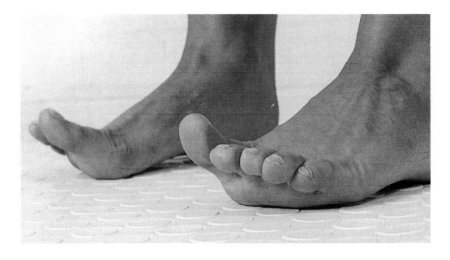

Left **Now lift your toes, keeping the balls of your feet on the floor, so that your weight is over the arches of your feet. Spread your toes and replace them on the floor, feeling the pads beneath each of them as you do so. Be conscious of your weight on your feet.**

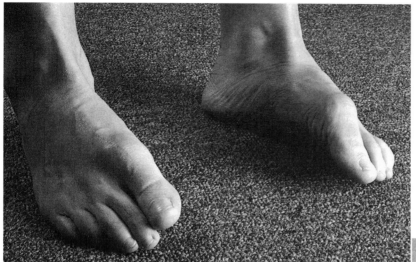

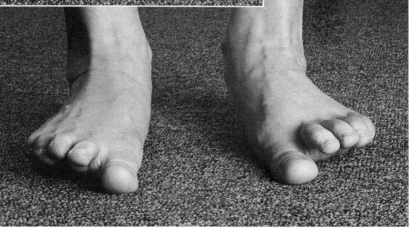

Left and below
Roll your weight from side to side, onto the outer and then the inner borders of the feet. If you roll very easily onto the inner edges, strengthen your arches by rolling onto the outer edges of your feet and walking a few steps.

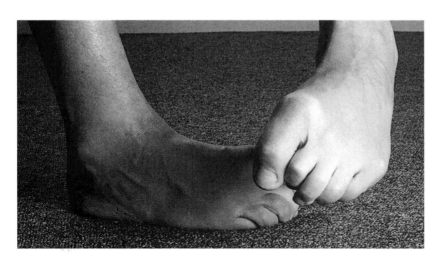

Left **Turn your feet inwards (pigeon toes) and again walk on the outer edges of your feet, lifting and placing one foot in front of the other.**

Right **Return to standing well balanced and, flattening your toes against the floor, pull them back towards your heels so that you feel a strong lift in the arches of your feet. Repeat this several times.
As an alternative, try picking up small objects such as pencils or marbles with your toes.**

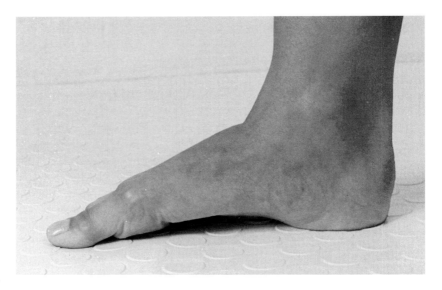

Massaging your feet with a ball

This is a wonderfully simple massage which can be done almost anywhere. All you need is a ball about the size of a squash ball.

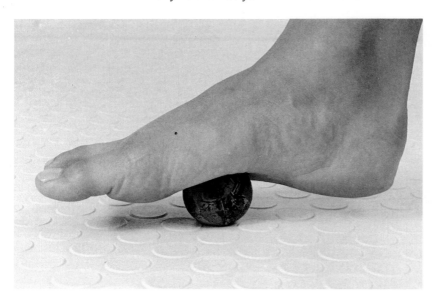

Left **Stand or sit comfortably, and place the ball underneath one of your feet. Imagine that the ball is covered with ink and that you are trying to get this ink onto the whole undersurface of your foot. Apply as much pressure as is comfortable.**

Repeat the process with the other foot, then take a minute to see how your feet feel. You may experience a tingling aliveness in your feet since the massage has reopened spaces between the small bones of the feet. You may notice certain places in your feet which are tender under the pressure of the ball. This could be due to the stimulation of certain of the reflex points of the feet.

Reflexology (zone therapy)

This is a very ancient system of treating the body through reflex points on the feet and hands. It is based on the belief that there are lines or channels of energy (meridians) which run through the body. For the purposes of reflexology, there are ten such meridians, which may be seen as running down from the head through the body, emerging at the five fingers and toes. Thus the hands and feet may be viewed as a map of the whole body, as seen on the chart.

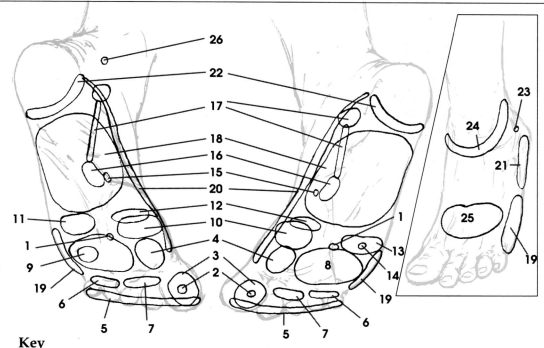

Key

1. Solar plexus and diaphragm
2. Pituitary gland
3. Brain
4. Thyroid and parathyroid gland
5. Sinuses
6. Ears
7. Eyes
8. Lungs
9. Heart (left foot only)
10. Stomach
11. Spleen (left foot only)
12. Pancreas
13. Liver (right foot only)
14. Gall bladder (right foot only)
15. Adrenal gland
16. Kidney
17. Bladder, ureter and urethra
18. Intestines
19. Arm and shoulder
20. Spine
21. Hip, thigh and leg
22. Sciatic nerve
23. Ovaries and testicles
24. Lymphatic system
25. Breasts
26. Uterus and prostate gland

Below **The action is
like a caterpillar
crawl. The pad of the
thumb is pressed into
the foot, and the
pressure rolls back
and then forward on
the ball of the thumb
which creeps
forward without
breaking contact.**

Reflex massage

Warm up each foot using brisk rubbing movements of the hands, which are held one on top and one underneath the foot. Loosen the ankles with several circles in each direction. Pull and waggle each of your toes and then massage systematically over each foot.

Since oil is too slippery, talc should be used when massaging your foot reflexes. There are two main ways of carrying out the massage; either perform thumb or finger petrissage over certain areas identified from the chart, or make progressive creeping pressures over the whole foot with the thumb.

There are also reflex points on the top of the feet which may be

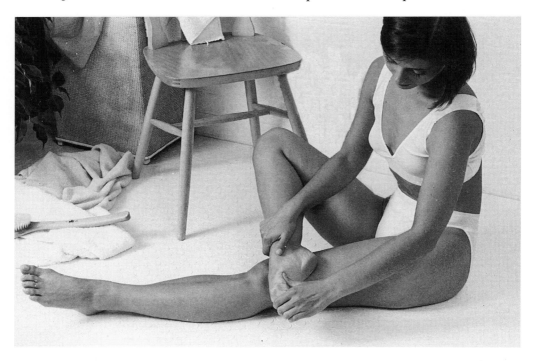

worked with the fingers, as may the lymphatic points on the ankle 'bracelets' (see p 71). The lymphatic system is a vital part of our immune defences. Since the lymph channels transport waste and toxins to the eliminating organs of the liver and kidneys, it is beneficial to work the reflex points for these organs, too. When working the kidney reflexes, start first with the bladder, then follow the ureter up to the kidney. In this way you clear the channels for elimination in the best order (see chart on page 67).

It is possible to buy sandals with little bobbles over the soles which massage and stimulate the foot reflexes as you walk.

Stretches for the feet

To some extent, ball massage will stretch the feet, since it opens up the spaces between the small bones. For other foot stretches, kneel on a padded surface.

Right **To stretch the front of the feet, kneel with your feet pointed back under you and your hands placed beside your knees. Taking your weight on your hands, roll back so that your knees lift off the floor and you feel the stretch in your shins and feet.**

Below left **Spread your toes wide to open spaces between them.**

Below right **Close and turn the toes under, squeezing to make knuckles across your feet. Repeat a few times.**

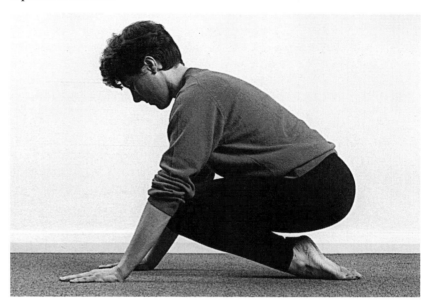

To stretch the arches of your feet and strengthen your toes, turn your toes under and sit back onto your heels. You can add more weight to the stretch by leaning back a little.

To stretch your toes, sit on the floor or in a chair, your feet resting on their heels.

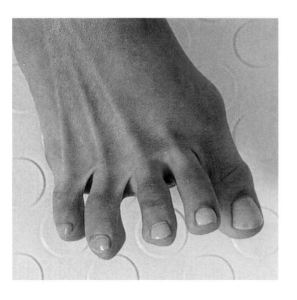

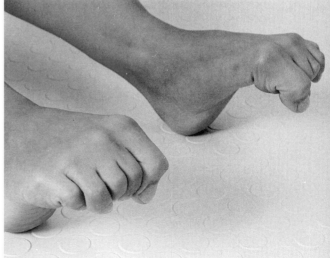

Adding a spring to your step with massage

This simple routine is designed to tone up and invigorate the muscles of the legs, and is particularly useful before an active day at work or at play. The same routine will revive tired muscles after a long, hard day or a strenuous exercise routine. Using essential oils will add to the pleasure of the massage, but remember that if you start with a bath or a shower, the water temperature should be relatively cool, since the therapeutic agents in the oils cannot be absorbed if you are perspiring.

What about varicose veins?

Avoid massage directly over a varicose vein, since this could dislodge small blood clots, giving rise to dangerous consequences. Massaging above the site of the varicose vein is harmless, and a very light stroking at the side of such veins may be practised if you have first consulted your doctor.

The leg routine

This may conveniently follow on after massaging the feet, although either massage may be done alone. You will need a towel, a pillow, one or two chairs and a massage oil or cream. For use of essential oils see pages 14 and 15.

Spread your towel on the floor and sit comfortably, bending one leg so that your foot is flat on the floor and the calf and thigh muscles are relaxed. Alternatively, sit on a chair with one leg bent and the foot resting on a second chair.

Right **Apply oil or cream to your hands and stroke it onto your lower leg. Make each movement several times.**

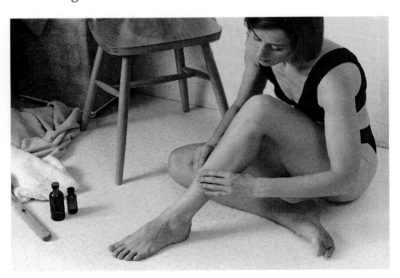

Right **Starting at the ankle and linking your thumbs behind the ankle, use the pads of your fingers to petrissage around the bracelet of the ankle.**

Inset **Continue the petrissage movements up on either side of the shinbone to the knee.**

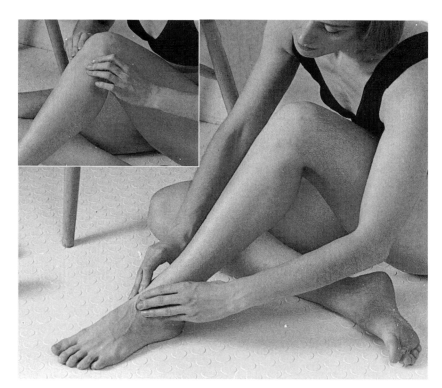

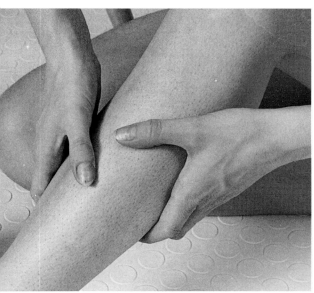

Left **Keeping both hands at the front of the shin, stroke lightly down to the ankle, turning the hands to pull back through the calf muscles towards the knee.**
Keeping the fingers cupped round the calf, slide them out through the muscle towards the thumbs with light pressure, then gently glide them back. Work up and down the calf in this way. With the hands held flat on either side of the calf muscle, wobble the calf until it becomes completely flaccid.

Straighten your leg slightly so that you can make large circles around the back of the knee with the fingers of alternate hands. Then, using the thumbs, petrissage all around the front of the knee, loosening the kneecap.

Thigh massage can be more vigorous, since the muscles are larger. So
1 Make kneading movements round the thigh, getting deep into the muscles in each area. Then, keeping hands and wrists relaxed, make loose fists and pummel the thighs.

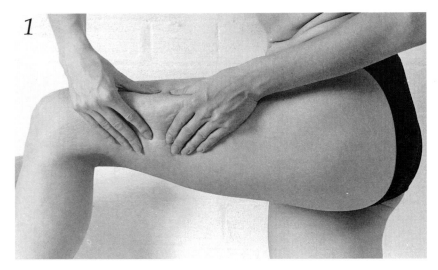

Alternatively, use cupped hands (*2*) or the sides of the hands (*3*) to make rapid cupping and hacking movements.

4 Finally, stroke the thighs, bringing the movements strongly up towards the lymph glands in the groin to encourage the dispersal of waste and toxins.

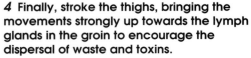

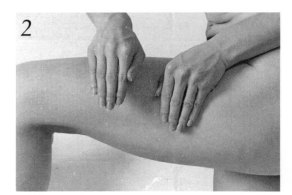

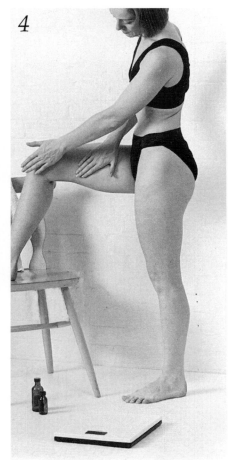

N.B .The movements just described will encourage circulation and cause a temporary reddening of the thighs, but should not be painful. They can be quite tiring to perform, however!

Perform the same sequence on each leg, then lie back on your towel, supporting your head and/or pelvis with a pillow if necessary. Bring your knees to your chest, hugging the legs in, then extend the legs upwards with bent knees ready for the 'jelly wobble'. Simply let go -- vibrate the legs, letting the muscles wobble and the joints shake free.

Dealing with cellulite

What is cellulite?

It is quite difficult to define cellulite accurately, although many authorities agree that fat is a constituent of it. Women are nevertheless often familiar with cellulite to a greater or lesser degree. Typically, it is an accumulation of lumpy, ridged flesh on hips and thighs which gives an 'orange peel' effect when pinched. Many medical experts believe that fat is fat and that that cellulite as a separate problem does not exist. Complementary and beauty therapists agree that fat is present, but that toxic wastes and water are also significant components, and that it is these which give the tissue its distinctive appearance.

Why are women so prone to cellulite?

Fat distribution and its storage in special cells of the body is governed by female hormones. In women, this distribution is centred on the hips, thighs and buttocks because the fat cells of tissues in these areas are particularly able to absorb fatty acids and conserve them; for this reason, fat is very difficult to lose in these areas.

How do we acquire cellulite?

Given the chance, the body does a pretty good job of neutralising and eliminating toxins. However, in our fast-moving, high-tech world we are exposed to more and more toxins, some of which we may choose to avoid and others about which we can do little. We thus have toxic waste cluttering up our circulatory systems, and it needs to be neutralised, excreted or buried away where it will do least harm.

When it is hidden away, however, it's rather like a lazy cleaner sweeping dust under a carpet or into a corner where it won't be noticed -- and you can probably guess where our bodies' dumping areas are! Fat cells, waste and a certain amount of water now get 'fenced in' by connective tissue in little pockets or bundles, thus creating the 'orange peel' effect.

What remedies are available?

Diet

Most diets won't eradicate cellulite completely, but a low fat or fat-free diet will help, as will a detoxifying diet consisting mostly of fruit and raw vegetables, with plenty of pure water to flush the toxins from the system. Natural diuretics such as fennel and celery also help, but coffee, although a diuretic, is said to be a contributing factor to the production of cellulite and should be avoided, as should alcohol.

Exercise

This improves circulation and can help to prevent the formation of cellulite. Cellulite under muscle can be very hard to shift, and some people believe that vigorous activity can actually increase its formation. Gentle exercise and stretching appears to be most beneficial.

Massage and aromatherapy

Opinions differ about whether massage for cellulite should be light or vigorous and deeply penetrating. My personal preference is for light massage with essential oils, allowing the therapeutic qualities of the oils themselves to do the hard work! Recipes for cellulite removal vary, but are made up from the oils described in the following section, with cypress and juniper being the most popular.

BEATING CELLULITE WITH ESSENTIAL OILS	
Cypress	Aids circulation and normalises female hormones
Juniper	Stimulates circulation and aids elimination of toxic wastes
Rosemary and lavender	Relieves lymphatic congestion
Geranium	Stimulates the lymphatic system and balances hormone production
Lemon	Decongests body and mind

Mix the oils of your choice in a suitable carrier oil (see page 15) and shake the bottle before use. My favourite oil, which also eases arthritic joints, is made up of rosemary and lavender (30 drops each), juniper (15 drops) and geranium (5 drops) in 200 ml of massage oil.

Before the massage, stimulate the lymphatic system by skin brushing, using a natural bristle brush. Starting with your limbs, brush upwards towards your heart, covering both sides of arms and legs and including the palms of your hands and the soles of your feet. Brush over your torso, front and back. The lymphatic channels are quite close to the surface of your skin, so pressure need not be so deep, though brushing may be as vigorous as feels comfortable. You will find that your skin benefits in texture and appearance from regular brushing. After the massage, finish by stimulating the lymphatic areas of your hands and feet, following the chart on p. 67.

Stretches for better-looking legs

Warm up and loosen your hips by doing some leg swings, holding onto the back of a chair for support. Swing your leg forwards and back from the hip, making the leg feel heavy and relaxed. Allow your knee to 'give' with the swing. Repeat on the other side.

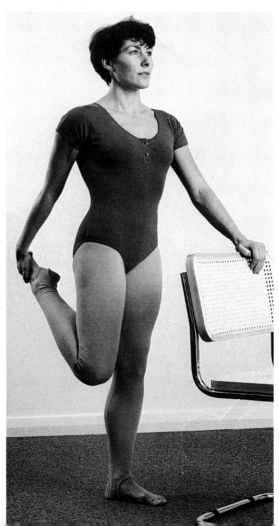

Right **With knees relaxed bring your right heel up to touch your bottom, holding it with your right hand. If you need more stretch, try to keep your knees together and straighten your left leg without allowing your bottom to poke out. Hold the stretch, then repeat with your left leg.**

75

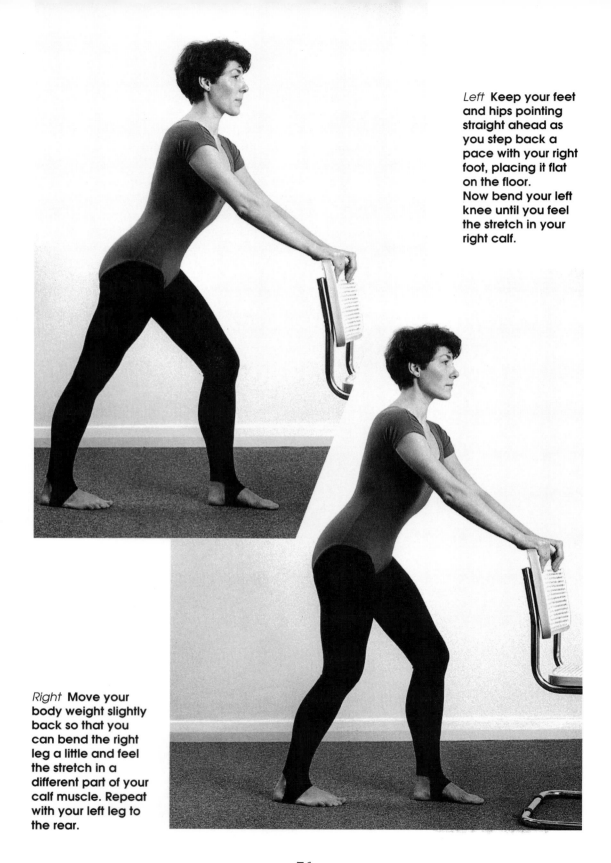

Left **Keep your feet
and hips pointing
straight ahead as
you step back a
pace with your right
foot, placing it flat
on the floor.
Now bend your left
knee until you feel
the stretch in your
right calf.**

Right **Move your
body weight slightly
back so that you
can bend the right
leg a little and feel
the stretch in a
different part of your
calf muscle. Repeat
with your left leg to
the rear.**

Right and below
With your right knee forward and aligned over your foot, lean forwards until you feel a stretch at the front of your hip and thigh.

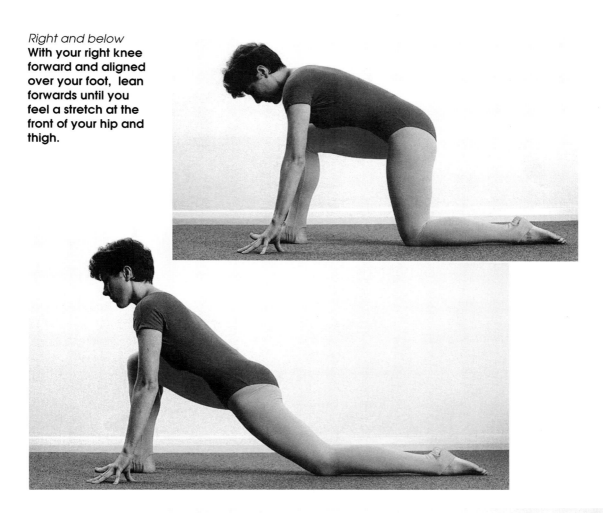

Right **To increase your stretch, tuck the toes of your left foot under, and push back on your heel until your knee lifts off the floor. Release the stretch and repeat on the other side.**

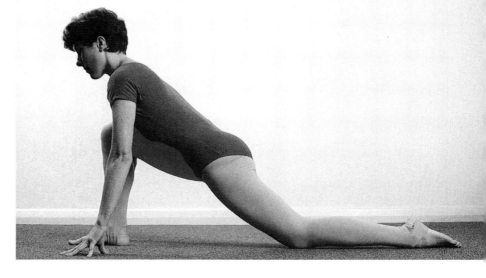

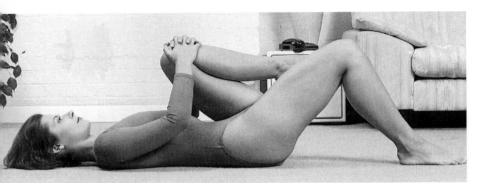

Left **Lying on your back, clasp your left knee to your chest, then extend your leg upwards, feeling the stretch at the back of your thigh. Massage the muscles, particularly at the back of the knee, to help soften and relax them.**

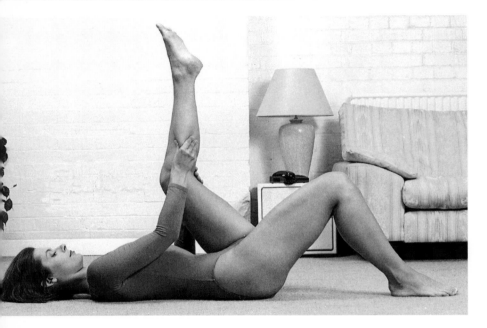

Right **To increase the stretch, gently limber the leg towards you.**

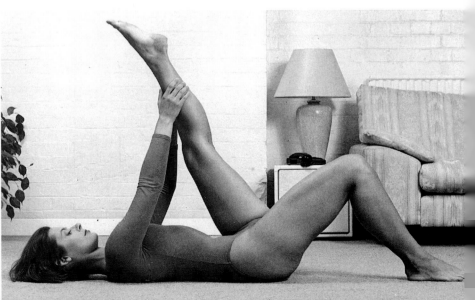

The above stretches will help to equalise the pull of the thigh muscles on the pelvis, giving better posture and freedom of movement. They are beneficial on their own, but especially so after massage, when the muscles are already relaxed and their stretch will be greater.

Routines to help your arms and hands

Unlike our feet, our hands are very much visible to ourselves and to others as we go about our daily lives, so we tend to take care of the way they look. We may be less careful, however, about maintaining their full mobility and flexibility and about minimising the chances of repetitive strain injury.

In order to make so many small intricate movements, the anatomy of the hand is quite complex, involving a number of small bones and joints, plus the tendons and ligaments which hold the structure together and keep it mobile. If we constantly repeat one particular movement, our tendons may become inflamed and swollen, causing pain. Rest, stretching and strengthening exercises minimise this risk.

Hand exercise and massage using a ball

You will need a ball about the size of an orange (or use an orange!). Sit comfortably erect and, holding the ball between your palms, roll it round and round, applying more pressure as necessary.

Left **Roll the ball for a few minutes to warm up.**

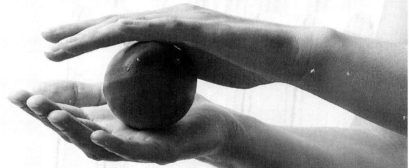

Right **Then roll it out along each finger and thumb in turn, applying sufficient pressure to bend them backwards as you roll.**

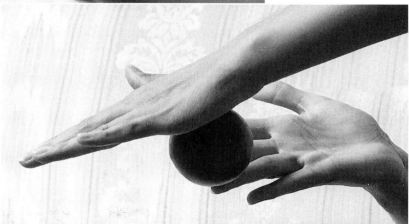

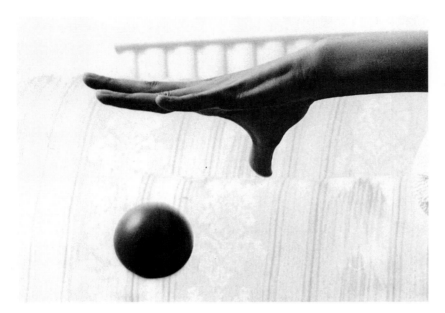

Left **Hold the ball in one hand as if about to bounce it on the floor. Exercise your fingers by releasing the ball, spreading your fingers wide and then catching the ball with a firm grip before it hits the ground.**

Hand exercise and massage using oil or cream

If you are in the habit of applying a hand cream, you can conveniently add some extra movements to your routine. If not, create some time for a little maintenance which will pay dividends.

Apply cream or oil to your hands, and rub them together to spread the massage medium. Link your fingers and rub your hands, both with palms together and with one hand over the other. With thumb petrissage movements, work into your wrists and then make several wrist circles in each direction.

Holding each finger in turn between the thumb and forefinger of the opposite hand, press along the sides and then along the back and front surfaces, working towards the fingertip each time. Do the same for the thumb.

Then, holding as before, make little twisting movements as you gently pull each of your fingers and thumbs. Repeat for the other hand and then make alternate fist-and-spread finger movements, squeezing and stretching several times. Finish by playing an imaginary piano, making sure all the fingers move.

Using your thumbs, massage the palm of each hand in turn. Make small petrissage or creeping movements to treat all the reflex points.

Using thumb creeping movements, work into the web and space between each of your fingers. Finish with soothing stroking movements, drawing the strokes over your wrists and onto your forearms so that your hands feel 'connected'.

Arm massage may conveniently follow on after massaging your hands, using the same oil or cream.

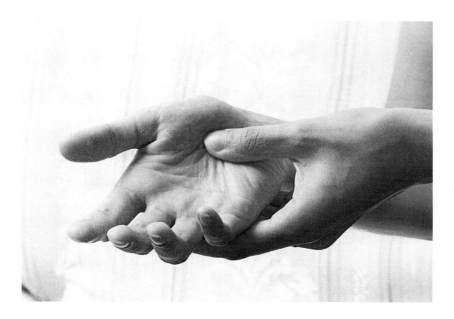

eft **Massage over the reflexology point on the palms of the hand with small petrissage movements.**

Right **Apply a little cream or oil to your arm, making long sweeping strokes up the inside and down the outside of the arm. Make the strokes stronger as they come towards your heart.**

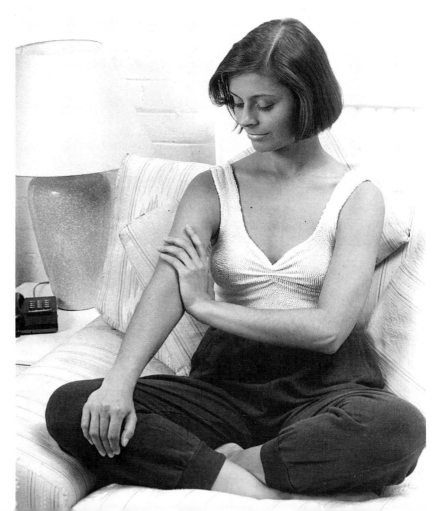

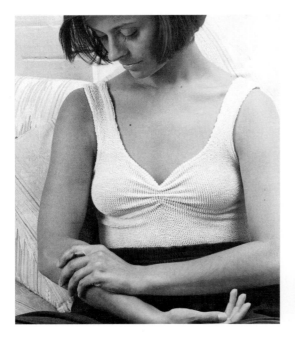

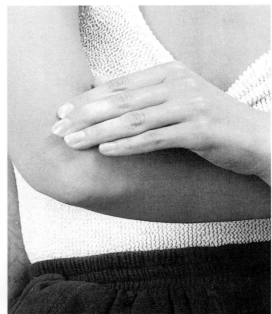

Above left **Make kneading and twisting movements over the muscles of your forearm and then work more deeply with your thumb, feeling for the spaces between the bones and the separation of the muscles.**

Above right **Make circling movements at the elbow, both on the inner and outer sides of your arm.**

Right **Make kneading and twisting movements into the muscles of your upper arm, and squeeze the muscles between your fingers and the heel of your hand. Use deeper petrissage movements as feels necessary. Finish with sweeping effleurage movements.**

Follow the massage with the shoulder stretches already described on page 21, since these will also work on the upper arm.

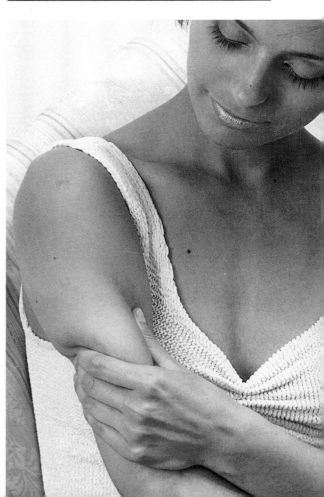

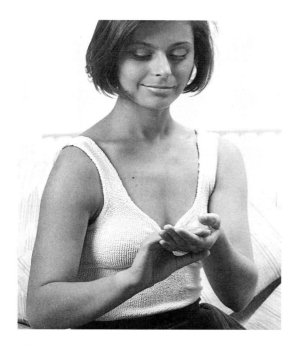

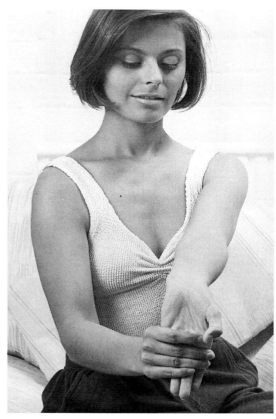

Above and right **To stretch the forearm and flex the wrist, hold your left hand in your right and fully extend both arms forward. At the same time, pull your left hand back to flex the wrist. Repeat for your right arm.**

Right **Next, turn your hands inwards, place them back to back and then draw your elbows downwards until you feel a good stretch in the back of your wrists. Clasp your hands together and circle your wrists in each direction. Lastly, reach up with your arms above your head and, as if trying to reach the ceiling, further extend one arm and then the other.**

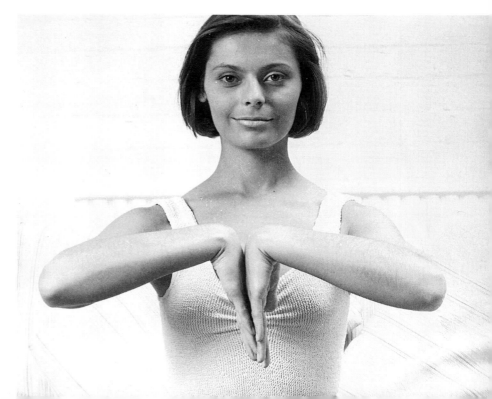

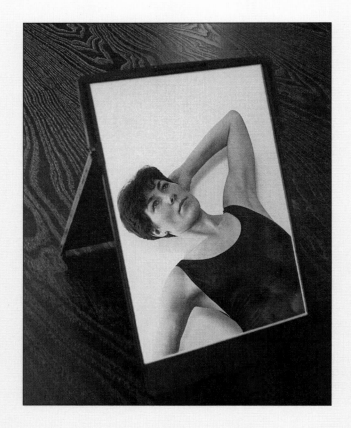

6

Here's looking at you

*Massage and exercise can help give
your face a new look*

It's the only one you've got!

Your face is the part of yourself that most represents what you choose to express to other people. Only a few people are expert at reading body language, but most are able to read a face to some degree or another, and whilst they would probably not attempt to make a diagnosis of your state of health -- as in some Eastern therapies -- they may accurately determine your mood. Though we may think of 'putting your best foot forward', how many expressions do we have about 'facing things'? For example: "put on a brave face/a bold face/ a happy face". There are songs to suggest painting a smile on your face and facing the music. You can probably think of more examples.

Window of the soul

The eyes also give clues to our whole state of being, and the many small muscles of the face give us our characteristic expressions -- and eventually our character lines. Even though the actual centre of the body lies just below the navel (if you doubt this, think about an acrobat or a trapeze artist balancing across a bar: the point at which the weight of the upper body balances that of the lower half lies somewhere just below the waist), it is not surprising that we become focussed and centred on the head and brain.

Reflection of the whole body

It is therefore natural that we should want to present the best face possible as we go about our lives. To do this, we must not only care about our skin with the many skin preparations that are available, but we must also take account of the stresses and strains of the whole body which are reflected in our faces and eyes. In the first section we will concentrate on releasing and relaxing tension rather than stretching, since the muscles and tissues with which we are dealing are particularly delicate. The massage techniques will appear later.

Facing up to your face

Before starting, take a moment to concentrate on your head and face. Is your head carried proudly and well balanced, or does your chin push forward, tilting your head back and shortening the back of your neck? Does the skin of your face feel soft and relaxed, or is it taut and tense? Is your facial expression fixed in a frown or a smile?

The head and posture

Start by sitting comfortably erect, and perform the 'triangle' visualisation outlined in chapter 3 (page 40) so that your neck is lengthened, your head lifted to the apex and your shoulders pulled down to the base angles of the triangle.

Now imagine your head at the top of your spine balanced at a point inside your skull at about the level of your ears. Feel the weight of your head by making gentle nodding movements as you keep the balance.

Checking for tension

Most of our facial tension comes from tightening the muscles of the jaw; try clenching your teeth for a moment and see what happens to your face and neck and also to your breathing.

Test how much unnecessary tension is going into your face and jaw. Admittedly, it might be somewhat anti-social to go around with your mouth hanging open, but the chances are that you are putting a lot of effort into keeping it shut!

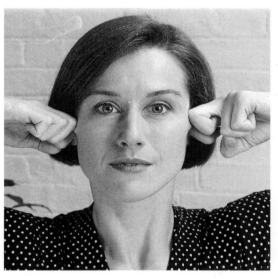

Left **Check the muscles at the hinge of your jaw; if you open and close your mouth you will feel this hinge point just in front of your ears. Place the knuckles of the first two fingers of your hand against the jaw hinge and then move them as if turning a screwdriver. If there is too much tension in these muscles, this movement will be painful.**

Below **Open your mouth as wide as possible in a silent scream . . .**
. . . or make very exaggerated "oo" and "ee" lip movements.
Alternatively, imagine chewing a really big toffee so that your mouth moves into positions that are different from your normal expression. When you stop, you should feel that your jaw has relaxed and that your cheeks feel soft and smooth.

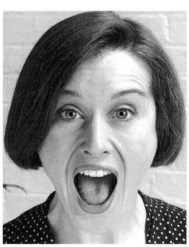
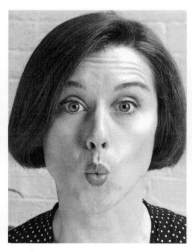
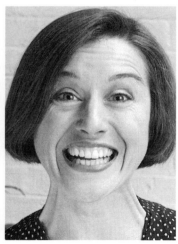

Breathing and tension release

Breathing exercises will also release tension in your face and, since they act to calm the mind as well, you get double benefit from trying them.

Sit or lie comfortably and take a moment to align your body so that you are breathing comfortably and easily. Take a deep breath and imagine blowing a feather away from your face as you breathe out through pursed lips. Keep your outbreath as steady as possible.

Take a deep breath as before. This time as you breathe out make a humming sound, keeping the sound steady for as long as possible. Do this a few times and experiment with the sound to see if you can make it resonate within the spaces of your face -- the mouth itself and the sinuses. If you are lying down, roll onto your side before sitting up.

However foolish it may seem, try punching a pillow really hard for a minute or two. This not only allows you to vent your feelings about the world around you (perhaps with suitable visualisations) but it is also good exercise as well as producing within you a very relaxed state.

Take a moment or two to observe how you feel. Does the balance of your head feel better than when you started? Does your face feel softer and fuller?

N.B. *If you want to follow on with a facial massage, you can skip the next section.*

Exercising and relaxing the eyes

These days, many of us spend time in front of a screen, watching TV or operating computerised equipment. Unless we take preventative measures, the consequences may be eye strain and postural fatigue. Many people are sensitive to the effects of VDU screens, and guidelines have been drawn up to minimise discomfort. These include:

> • **Placing the screen away from the direct light of a window.**
>
> • **Making sure that your chair is high enough, so that you look downwards at the screen.**
>
> •**Taking frequent short breaks and making opportunities to stretch and move around.**

Alternative remedies

There are also alternative remedies. For instance, to neutralise any effects of working in front of a VDU screen, try taking equal doses of the salts Kali Mur and Nat Mur. These biochemical tissue salts can be obtained from your local health shop. These have no side-effects and may be taken as often as every half hour.

You can also use essential oil of Rosemary to aid concentration. A drop of the oil may be placed on a tissue or onto a light bulb, or you may use a special burner to disperse the fragrance into the air.

The eye workout

Most of the methods for improving eyesight make great use of relaxation methods. One of the quickest and easiest is to splash water over the eyes, alternating a cold and warm splash. This may nevertheless not always be practical, especially if you are wearing eye make-up! Simply blinking the eyes has a refreshing effect, as does yawning. Both momentarily bring a slight watering to the eyes, which cleanses the surface.

Your eyes are controlled by a complicated system of muscles, some of which actually move the eye whilst others act to change the focus and the amount of light admitted. Like any other group of muscles, they become tired with over-use and stiff with under-use. These exercises will help:

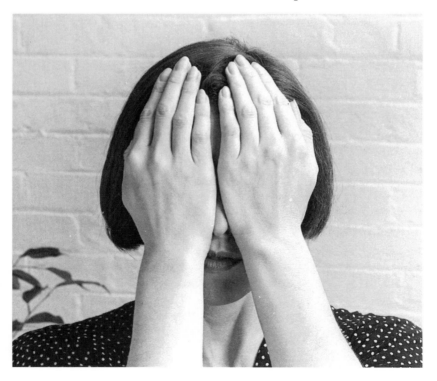

Before beginning, and in between the exercises, rest and relax the eyes completely by palming. This is done by covering the eyes with the palms of your hands so as to exclude light completely. Keep your eyes open under your palms and remain in this position for several minutes. In order to stay relaxed, it may be helpful to sit in front of a table so that you can rest your elbows.

Sitting comfortably upright and without moving your head, turn your eyes to look up and down several times. Then palm to rest. Continue the exercises, looking to right and left and up and down on each diagonal. Palm the eyes when you need to rest.

With your eyes make slow circles in each direction, trying not to leave out any part of the circle. Finally, choose two points, one in the distance and one close to you, and allow your focus to change from near to distant and back several times.

Rest your eyes well by palming for several minutes. You may find that things look brighter and clearer afterwards.

The do-it-yourself facial

Our skin is one of our most important organs, since it acts both as a protective covering and as a means of eliminating toxins. When, for one reason or another, the bodily systems become overloaded, we often suffer from skin complaints as accumulated toxins are pushed out to the surface. The skin of the face is particularly vulnerable, and rapidly shows the effects of too little sleep or too much good living.

Giving yourself a regular facial massage adds to the value of a good diet, rest and exercise in keeping your skin supple and clear of congestion. Add the 'face-lift' visualisation (see page 94) and you will be ready to face anything! This routine can easily follow your normal cleansing process; all you will need is a massage oil or cream, a soft clean flannel and possibly a headband. The movements are a combination of small pressures followed by gentle stroking, and act to stimulate the removal of toxins by the lymphatic circulation.

Cleaning the channels

Start with a well-cleansed face and neck; then, wringing out your flannel in hot water, place it over your face for a few moments. Next, apply sufficient oil or cream to allow your fingers to glide over the surface of your skin.

Below left and right
Clear the lymph drainage channels by making long stroking movements which start at the side of the neck, just below the ear. Sweep the fingers down, crossing the chest and finishing at the opposite armpit. Use alternating hands, the right hand stroking the left side of your neck and vice versa.

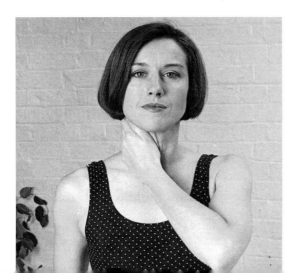
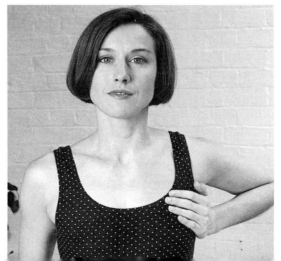

Don't press too hard here; the lymphatic circulatory system lies quite close to the surface, and the idea is to move any congestion outwards to the clearing channels.

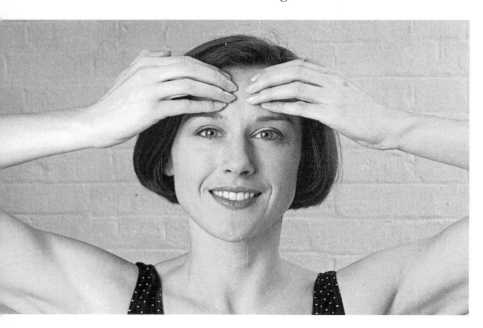

Left **Start from the top of your face and work downwards. Place your fingers at the centre of your forehead and apply gentle pressure. Repeat this several times, moving your fingers outwards a little each time until you reach your temples.**

Right **Make small rotating movements at your temples, then return to the original position, pressing your fingertips against your forehead and then sliding the fingers outwards to the temples.**

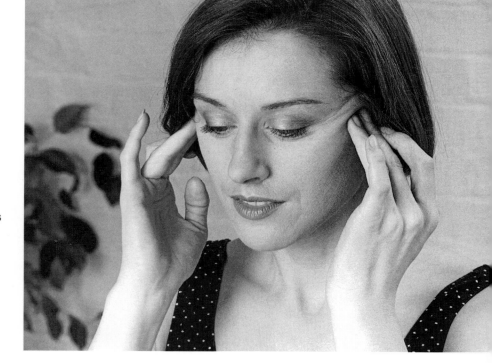

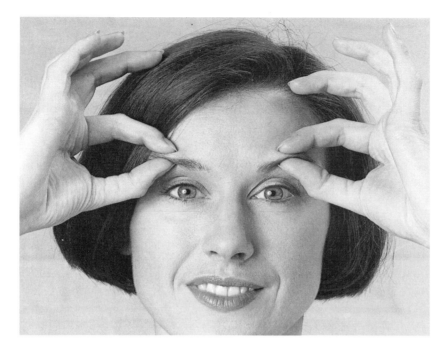

Left **Using your forefingers and thumbs, make little pinches all the way along the length of your eyebrows, then circle at the temples again.**

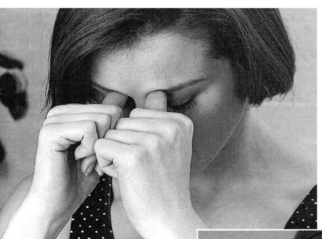

Left **Use pressure to relieve eye strain and brighten the eyes. Work on the inner part of the eye socket, press upwards towards the eyebrows with your thumbs.**

Right **Press down and inwards towards the nose with your fingers.**

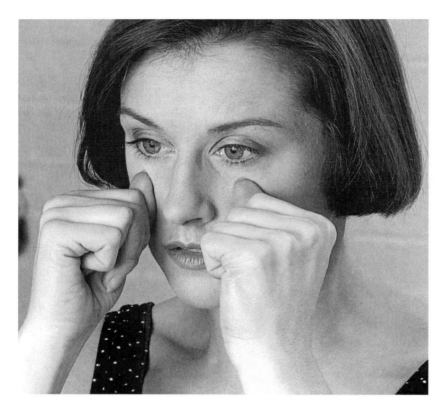

Left **Using the backs
of your thumbs,
work outwards from
your nose across
your cheekbones to
the front of your
ears. Make finger
circles at the hinge
point of the jaw and
then move on to
make circles over
your ears. Massage
your ears, imagining
unrolling all the
curled-over bits and
then making small
pinching and pulling
movements on
them. Finish by
gently pulling
downwards on your
earlobes.**

Right **With fingers
held apart, place
them on your face
level with your
nostrils. Apply gentle
pressure, then,
moving the fingers
outwards little by
little, continue
applying pressure
until you reach your
ears.**

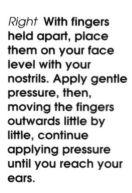

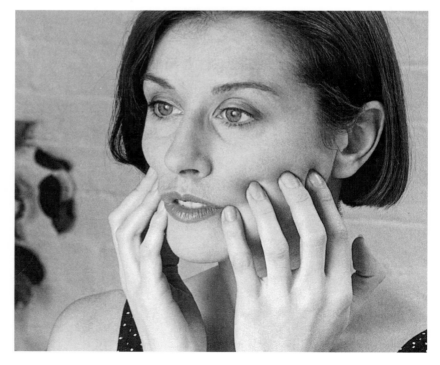

Carry out the same sequence of movements but this time starting from the sides of your mouth: then, from the centre of your chin, always working outwards. In the same three zones apply light pressure and then slide the fingers outwards.

Next, starting with your fingertips held just below your ears, make small finger circles down the sides of your neck, finishing at your collar bone.

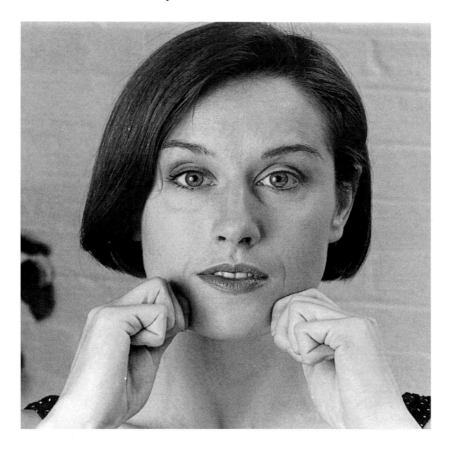

Left **Make firm pinching movements along the chin from the centre to the ears. Next, placing your hands lightly on your face with fingers at your hairline, gently draw them down the length of your face. Finish with the neck stroking movements that began the massage.**

End as you began

Use a flannel wrung out in hot water for a few moments as at the beginning of the routine, followed by a tissue to absorb excess cream or oil. Repeat, followed by wringing out the flannel in cold water and applying as before.

Now is the ideal time to carry out the relaxation and visualisation for the face described below, although it is so simple that it can be done at almost any time. You can record the instructions yourself with suitable background music and use the tape in your personal stereo during journey times.

The face-lift visualisation

Give yourself five or ten minutes of uninterrupted time space to do this.

Lie on your back with knees bent as in 'Back to Basics' (chapter 3, page 31), or sit comfortably erect with your feet flat on the floor and your hands relaxed. Take several deep breaths, allowing yourself to feel heavier and more relaxed with every outbreath. Allow your eyelids to become heavier until you gently close your eyes.

Scalp and forehead

Now concentrate your attention on the top of your head and the skin of your scalp. If it feels tight, imagine flattening your ears against the sides of your head, and feel the scalp relax.

Shift the concentration to your forehead. If it feels tight, raise your eyebrows up and down a few times. Now stop, and feel the smooth breadth of your forehead. Imagine your brow being stroked by cool, gentle fingers. Concentrate upon the space between your eyebrows and feel as if it is getting wider and wider; your eyebrows feel as if they are longer.

Raising your eyebrows

Now think about the arch of your right eyebrow: feel the curve of your right eyebrow as it lifts up and over from beside your nose outwards towards your ear. Think about your right eye under the arch of its brow, and imagine your right eye becoming larger and wider. Do the same for the arch of your left eyebrow and for your left eye.

Cheeks and jawline

Think about your cheeks and imagine them smooth and rounded as a baby's. Feel the soft fullness of your cheeks. Check that your teeth are not clenched together, and that your lips are soft and slightly parted. If you feel tense in the jaw, try the "oo" and "ee" exercise described at the beginning of this chapter. To lift the muscles of the jaw, imagine pulling and scraping your hair back and up towards the top of your head as if making a pony-tail.

Breathe in your favourite colour

Rest, concentrating on your breath and noticing the coolness of the air you breathe in. Feel it in the spaces of your nostrils, your mouth, throat and chest. Feel the warmer air of your outbreath and imagine it drawing out tightness, tension and toxins from your body. If you have a favourite colour, you may like to imagine breathing it in to fill all the parts of your body.

Aromatherapy for your face

The use of essential oils can add a really luxurious feeling to your facial massage. Choose a light carrier oil such as Sweet Almond, or the penetrating and nourishing Jojoba (in reality a wax) and add appropriate essential oils. If you want to improve the keeping quality of your oil, add a few drops of wheatgerm oil to the carrier oil before adding the essential oil of your choice. For guidelines on mixing oils, read the section in chapter 1 (page 15). You might like to try some of the following:

Oils of Rose, Jasmine or Neroli have a heady, lasting fragrance and are justly renowned in the realms of feminine beauty. They are nevertheless expensive, so you may want to find a reputable supplier who retails a ready-mixed facial oil of good quality.

Oil of Sandalwood is a good unisex oil which is soothing to the skin and can be particularly helpful if you suffer from dry skin and/or redness.

Oils of Lavender and Geranium are the balancers and harmonisers of aromatherapy. Geranium may be used to balance the skin's own oiliness.

Frankincense is an exotic oil uplifting to the spirits and to the mature skin.

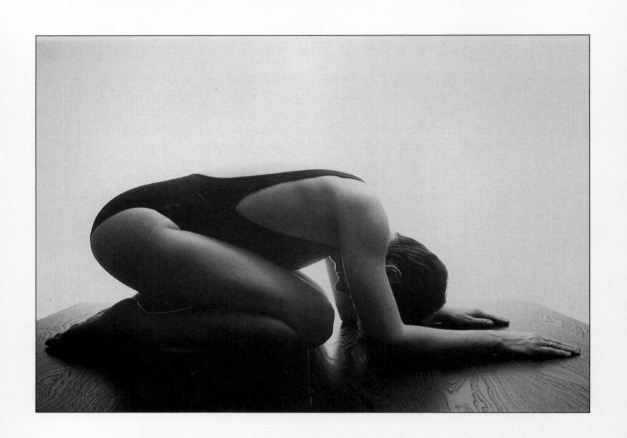

7
All of you

Whole-body routines, both for massage and stretching, ways of improving lymphatic circulation and 'washing the blues away' with aromatherapy.

Going with the flow

These routines include those which will take only a few minutes as well as those for the occasions when you can forget the clock and devote time to yourself alone. If you are short of time, one of the best things you can do for your health and for your skin is to stimulate the lymph and blood circulation by dry-brushing your skin before you have a bath or shower.

What is the lymphatic system?

The lymphatic circulation (mentioned previously in the section on cellulite, page 73) is part of the immune system and is thus one of the most important systems for maintaining health. It is the main highway of the body's defence and cleansing system and consists of a network of vessels running throughout the body in much the same way as the blood is circulated. Within the lymph channels, fluid transports waste for disposal and carries the immune defence cells of the body. These cells, called lymphocytes, are important because they have the ability to recognise harmful agents, such as viruses and certain bacteria, and produce antibodies which destroy them.

Unlike the blood system, however, the lymphatic circulation has no pump, and the fluid is kept flowing through the network by the action of our muscles. If we remain static for any length of time, fluid ceases to flow freely and can build up in the tissues, causing puffiness and swelling. Lack of movement can also cause the dumping of the toxin load in the congested area. Massage, including reflexology and aromatherapy, combined with exercise, is useful in dispersing any build up of fluid.

Dry skin brushing

Once you have made this a part of your normal body-cleansing routine, you will notice such a great improvement in the softness and clarity of your skin that you will easily keep up the habit. All you need is a large brush made of natural bristle -- and a little energy.

Before you take a bath or shower, brush your body all over, starting from the soles of your feet and working upwards over your legs and over the front and back of your body. Always work in the direction of your heart, and use as much pressure as feels comfortable. Do the same for your hands and arms, your shoulders and the back of your neck. Stimulate your scalp if you wish, but avoid brushing over your face.

Brushing will get rid of waste matter on your skin and make its elimination function more efficient; it will also encourage the dispersal of cellulite, and is environmentally friendly in that you need to use less soap or shower gel.

Reflex massage for your lymphatic system

This takes just a few minutes at the end of your bath or shower.

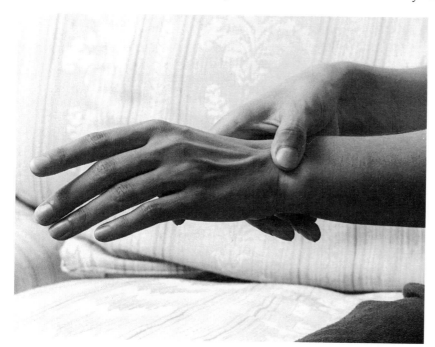

Left **Using little thumb circles, massage into the 'bracelet' creases of each wrist.**

Right **Then massage into the ankle 'bracelets' in the same way, using circling movements with all of your fingers.**

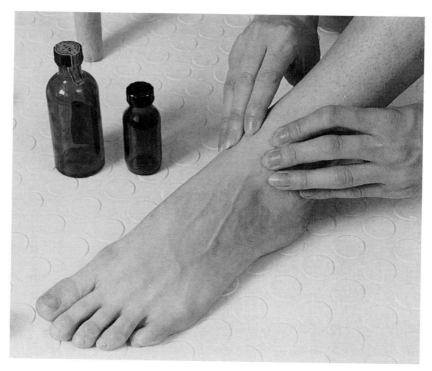

Stimulating strategies

If you are in need of a little extra 'zing' to your day, follow skin brushing with a cold shower, or use one of the following routines.

Tapping and rapping

Massage can be used to stimulate and invigorate as well as to soothe and relax. If you need a quick energiser, try using an all-over slapping and rapping technique that derives from an Oriental system called Do-in.

Sit or stand comfortably and start by rubbing and clapping your hands together to bring energy into your hands. Next, try rapping down the side of your neck and out along your shoulder with a loose fist. Carry on with these movements down the inside of your arm and up the outside to your shoulder. Repeat the movements using more force if it feels necessary, then do the other side.

Now lean forward and, reaching up behind your back as high as possible, make percussive movements downwards along either side of the spine and onto each buttock.

Coming back to an upright position again, continue the movements down the inside of the legs and up the outside, returning to the buttocks once more.

Next make rapping movements up your body, over your chest and onto your breast bone just below the collar bones. Think about those old Tarzan movies and make a noise too if you feel like it -- it's great as a start to the day, even if it amazes the neighbours! This movement stimulates your thymus gland, an important part of the immune system.

Finally, make tapping and rapping movements all over your head to wake up your brain.

Friction with a towel

Other stimulating strategies include the skin brushing and cold shower options already described, and a cool bath using uplifting essential oils (see page 102). The use of a friction towel is also helpful. These towels are made from coarse linen fibres and act upon the skin in a similar way to skin brushing.

Cooling everything down

When you really want to unwind, it's time to pull out all the stops, adding every bit of comfort and luxury to your all-over massage, which can be done without any preliminaries, or following a warm, relaxing bath. If you are using essential oils in your massage, use complementary oils in your bath to make the routine one big scented

treat. If you are short of time, you can use a ~~~~~~~~
own, followed by a few massage strokes as yo~ ~~~~ ~ody lotion, or
you may treat your whole body through your feet (see section on
reflexology, page 67).

Set the scene

Create a pleasant space in which to undertake your massage:
sometimes candlelight creates the right mood, whilst at other times,
covering a lamp (obviously not too near the bulb) with a coloured
scarf, or using a coloured bulb can be effective. Use music, incense
and any other props you can think of. Prepare in advance: you may
want to lie down to stretch and relax after the massage, so spread a
large towel or a blanket over something soft to lie on, and have
something warm nearby (which doesn't matter if it gets massage oil
on it!) in case you cool down more than you would have liked. Have
tissues and kitchen paper handy, ready to absorb any excess oil or
cream.

Place your massage medium at hand; you may want to use talc on
your feet and oil or lotion on your body. Perhaps you will want to
use a different oil for your face than for the rest of the massage, or
you may want to use an anti-cellulite oil or cream over your thighs.
Have all these things ready and within reach so that you don't have
to break the flow of your massage once you start.

The massage

Now you can 'go to town' and use all your favourite strokes from
each section. Decide on the order of your massage; for instance you
may want to start with a facial, then continue downwards onto your
neck, shoulders and arms, following these with your abdomen,
back, legs and finally your feet. Be relaxed, and don't try to
remember all the strokes and sequences; just follow the logical
progression through your body. Experiment a little to find what feels
right, and you will find that although you may leave out certain
strokes, your ultimate bodily feeling will be one of wholeness and
completeness. If you really can't bear to leave out a single stroke,
write notes for yourself or record the sequence of strokes onto a tape
to play back while you work.

Allow yourself a period of relaxation, or even sleep, at the end of
your massage, covering yourself with an extra towel or blanket to
keep warm and comfortable.

Last things

To complete the whole massage programme, wash your hands under
running water to remove any oil or lotion on them and also to

...n re...e any negative vibrations you may have picked up. Drink a glass of water or fruit juice to help disperse any toxins through your excretory system.

You may wish to incorporate stretch routines as you proceed through your massage, or you may save them until the end. Whatever your choice, you can perform some of the stretch routines outlined at the end of this chapter (pages 104 108).

Washing the blues away

Water is a great cleanser, both in actuality and symbolically. If you have a special massaging showerhead or have access to a jacuzzi, you can utilise the properties of water in your own hydrotherapy massage, selecting the intensity of the water jets according to the degree of tension in your muscles. In any event, you can use aromatherapy oils in your bath as a simple and completely effortless body-treat. When you use essential oils in your bath, there are three things to remember:

> • **The oils are volatile and will rapidly vaporise, therefore they should be added to a drawn bath for maximum effect.**
>
> • **Absorption of the therapeutic agents cannot occur whilst you are eliminating through the skin (sweating), so your bath water should be comfortably warm, not hot.**
>
> • **The absorption will continue for a period of time after your bath.**
>
> • **When adding essential oils to your bath, use a total of 8-10 drops of oil, which may be a single oil or a mixture of oils. (Note: if you have a sensitive skin, or when using essential oils in a bath for children, it is best to dilute the oils in a carrier oil before adding to the bath.)**

Disperse the oil by agitating the water with your hands. This creates a film of tiny droplets all over the surface of the water, and as you enter the bath your body will become coated with a film of oil. Relax in the bath for ten to fifteen minutes, enjoying your chosen aroma and allowing the therapeutic agents to be absorbed into your body tissues. Afterwards wrap yourself up in a soft towel or bathrobe and simply pat yourself dry.

AROMATHERAPY FOR THE BATH

Muscle fatigue	Rosemary Lemongrass Lavender Marjoram
Mental fatigue	Rosemary Basil
Cleansing and detoxifying	Juniper Rosemary Lavender Geranium Lemon
Diuretic and anti-cellulite	Juniper Cypress Sweet fennel Rosemary Geranium
Uplifting and anti-depressant	Clary sage Bergamot Geranium Melissa Patchouli
Aphrodisiac	Ylang ylang Rose Neroli Jasmine
Sedative and soporific	Lavender Camomile Neroli Sandalwood

Stretching it out

Putting all our joints through their full range of movement once a day plays an essential part in keeping active and mobile throughout life. By stretching, we help to spread the natural wear and tear evenly round joints and minimise such problems as arthritis. These days, most people are very much aware of the need to take regular exercise, in particular, aerobic exercise which maintains heart and lung efficiency.

However, we should not forget in our eagerness to get going that stretching is an important part of the warm-up and warm-down phase of physical activity. Our bodily strength, stamina and suppleness may decline gradually with age, but flexibility, once gained, declines more slowly than other aspects of fitness..

The two minute stretch

Make stretching part of your wake-up routine; it feels such an easy and natural thing to do, and will really get your day off to a good start. You can even stretch in bed, but it's better done on the floor. However, if you do decide to stretch in bed, or just after you get up, you won't need to perform warm-up exercises, since your body will be warm already. Bring your arms back to lie beside your body and imagine that you could make six holes in the floor or in your mattress using the back of your head, both elbows, your tail bone and both heels. Inhale, and as you exhale, push to make the six holes, inhale and totally let go.

Lie flat on your back and stretch your arms up over your head. Take a deep breath and, as you exhale, stretch your legs right down to the tips of your toes and your arms to the tips of your fingers. Inhale and relax everything. Repeat two or three times, really extending your body. I call this one 'the rack' because it really elongates you!

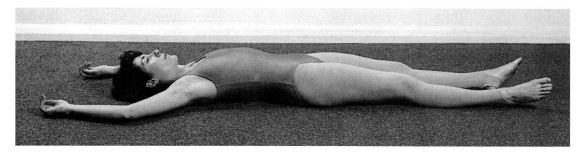

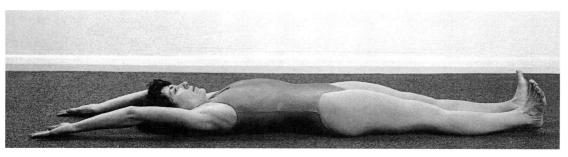

The four-part stretch routine

If you wish to devote more time to stretching, you could use this two-minute stretch at the end of a longer routine.

For this routine, work through the body in four sections: (1) the neck, shoulders and arms; (2) the back and sides; (3) the hips and thighs, and (4) the lower legs and feet. You will find all the stretches described in the appropriate sections of this book, so what follows is a brief reminder to suggest just one way of putting together a whole-body routine. Warm up first, put on some music and dance or jog on the spot -- or take the easy option and have a hot shower! Whatever you use as a warm-up should be continued until you begin to perspire slightly.

1) Neck, shoulders and arms

Do a few shrugs and shoulder circles before beginning these stretches.

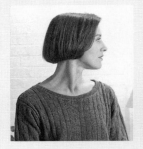 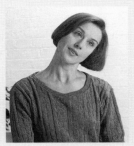 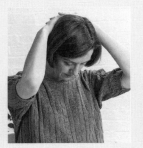 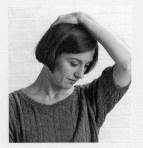

Turning head from side to side (page 44)   **Ear to shoulder (page 44)**   **Chin to chest (page 45)**   **Diagonal stretch (page 46)**

Below are all on page 21

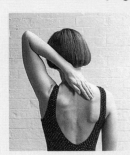 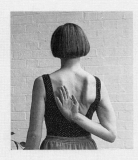 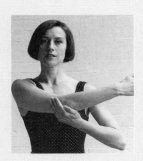 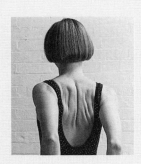

Hand to opposite shoulderblade behind head   **Hand to opposite shoulderblade behind back**   **Arm across body**   **Shoulder squeeze**

1) Neck, shoulders and arms (continued)

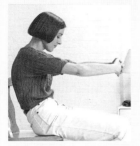 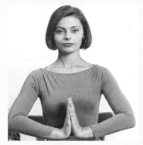 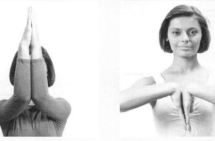

**Rounded-back
hand push
(page 46)**

**Prayer hands -- press and lift elbows
(page 22)**

**Back of wrist stretch
(page 83)**

2) Back and sides

Standing stretches

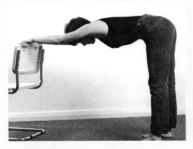 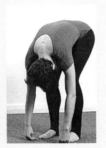 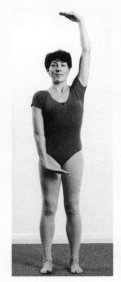

**Table stretch
(page 27)**

**Hanging loose
(page 28)**

**Side bend
(page 35)**

Left **Pushing hands
side stretch
(page 27)**

2) Back and sides (continued)

Kneeling on all fours

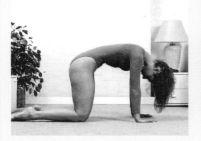

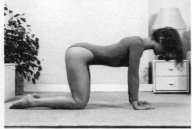

Cat stretch (page 29)

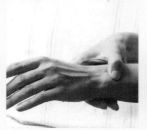

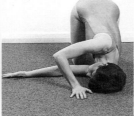

Threading the needle (page 30)

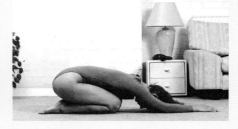

Pose of a child (page 30)

Lying with knees bent

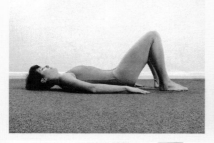

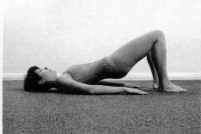

Left **Pelvic tilt, roll up through spine (page 31)**

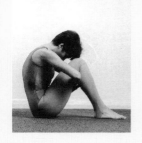

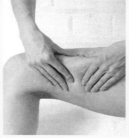

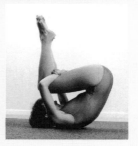

Left **Rock and roll (page 26)**

3) *Hip and thigh stretches*

Standing

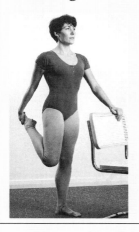

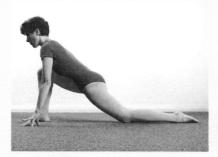

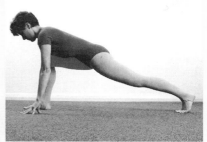

Left **Heel to bottom (page 75)**

Lunge stretch for groin (page 77)
Hips drop to side (not illustrated)
(page 30 for description)

Seated on floor

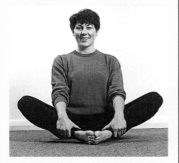

Inner thigh stretch (Introduction)

Lying supine

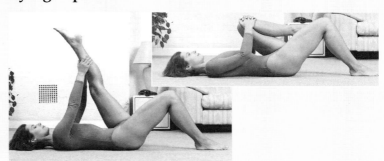

Knee to chest and limber (page 78)

4) *Lower legs and feet*

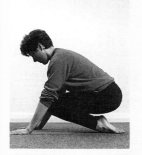

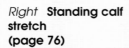

Left **Sitting on heels, knee lift (page 69)**

Right **Standing calf stretch (page 76)**

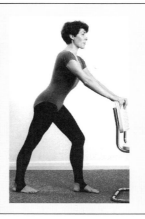

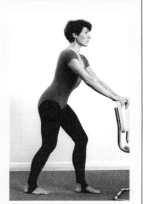

Epilogue

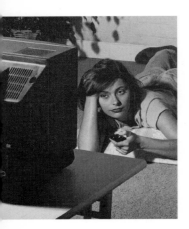

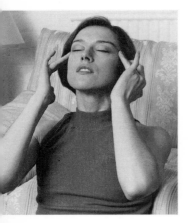

The techniques of self-massage and stretching are of course only part of a whole range of techniques available to anyone who wishes to 'look good, feel good', as the the classic phrase has it. Not all of us, however, can get to general fitness classes or to the newer trends of callanetics, cardiofunk or step workouts. 'Touching and stretching' is nevertheless so much designed for your quiet moments at home, that many of the exercises can easily be fitted into your everyday life without becoming a trial. The unconcious eye-strain induced by watching your favourite TV programme or reading can soon be relieved by facial massage techniques: the almost inevitable crunched-up postures we assume while working only stress us if we omit a few of the stretches that gently take our bodies back into shape. Touching and stretching are the *natural* ways of balancing the stresses that life inflicts upon us.

Yet, that being said, it is not a bad thing to remember the 'back-up' rules which allow our bodies the best chance of functioning well. Believe it or not, there are still a number of women down at my favourite fitness centre who work through an hour's fitness class, then change into their ordinary clothes and light a cigarette as they leave the building: there are also men who 'pump iron' or sweat buckets on an exercise bicycle before spending the evening at their favourite hostelry putting back more empty calories than they have shed a few hours earlier. I therefore have no compunction about reminding you (or maybe nagging at you) to back up your quest for relaxed fitness by looking at the things which *detract* from the look-good-feel-good aim. Most of the tips are contained in my friend Gloria Klein's book 'Face Up', but she says so much of what I would say on the subject that I'll let Gloria's words do the honours. . .

Smoking

The first thing you must do (if you haven't already done so) is to give up smoking completely. Smoking is not only bad for your health, but is fatal for your looks. Remember too that if you smoke, an alarming percentage of your red cells are carrying a deadly gas (carbon monoxide) rather than life-giving oxygen. Sure, there are a million excuses, but there is still no question about it -- if you are serious about maintaining your health and looks -- stop smoking!

Alcohol

Hurrah -- I don't have to be a *total* killjoy here, for there is some evidence that moderate amounts of alcohol may actually be good for you! The trouble for some folk is that moderate means no more than two units of alcohol (two glasses of wine, say) per day, and try to leave two days a week clear of alcohol. Recent studies have shown that women are particularly in danger of damaging their livers on smaller amounts of alcohol than men. So let me repeat this, because it is important. Alcohol in small amounts may relax you, improve your digestion and may even protect you from heart disease. But in larger amounts it is extremely dangerous, especially for women. If you are pregnant, or plan to be, cut alcohol out completely.

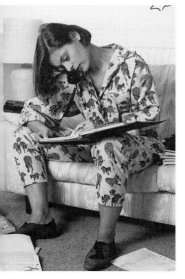

Sleep

Sleep is a great healer and rejuvenator. We need sleep to refresh and revive our bodies and our minds. When you are in a peaceful sleep, your heartbeat and digestion slow down, your blood pressure falls slightly and your breathing gets shallower. All these factors help to keep us healthy -- but the important point is that your body *needs* sleep time because in this state it is in the best position to repair damaged tissue, produce antibodies to fight infection and carry out many other health-maintaining processes. We even need to dream, even if we don't remember the results: people deprived of dream sleep become tense, irritable and confused. Sleeping pills suppress dream sleep and thus accelerate the slide to anxiety and depression.

Aspirins, tranquillizers and other drugs

It may be something of a media phrase to say that we have become a nation of pill-poppers; yet even if we are not, it may only be because of the high cost of all but the humble aspirin. The same media have nevertheless begun to alert us quite well to the fact that sleeping pills and tranquillizers can be not only physically dangerous but psychologically dangerous as well, since you can become addicted to them. Some of the blame for our pill-popping belongs to drug companies who market their products perhaps over-vigorously, and to doctors who use a prescription as an easy way out of having to listen to what is really bothering the patient. Yet as adults we must take some responsibility for the care of our bodies, and not insist on having a 'magic' pill when proper food and a few days' rest (partners and children permitting!) can make you well.

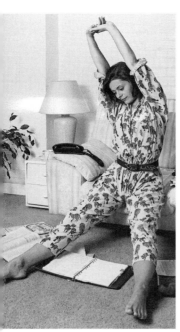

And finally . . .

. . . may I express the hope that you will find the self-massage and stretch routines easy and enjoyable to carry through. Never think of them as a rigid ritual which you *must* try to fit in every day. They are there to make you feel better -- and that means happier!

FRONT VIEW

1 **Pectoralis major** *(moves shoulder)*

2 **Biceps** *(bends and rotates forearm)*

3 **Serratus anterior** *(supports shoulder)*

4 **External oblique** *(supports and bends spine)*

5 **Rectus abdominis** *(supports abdomen)*

6 **Sartorius** *(rotates and bends leg)*

7 **Quadriceps** *(straighten leg)*

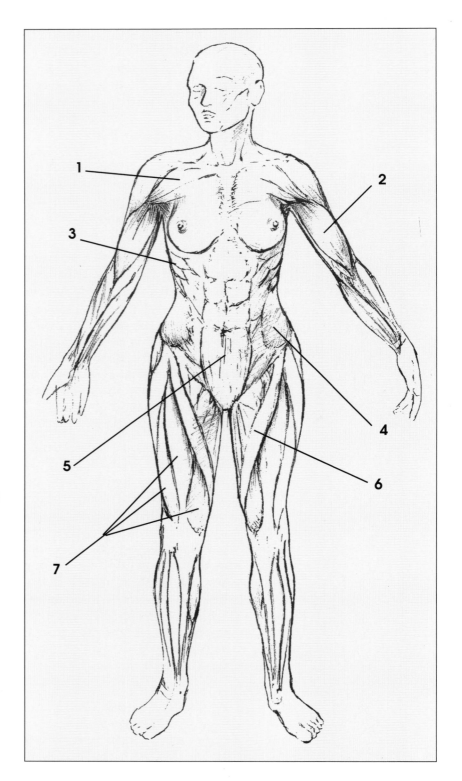

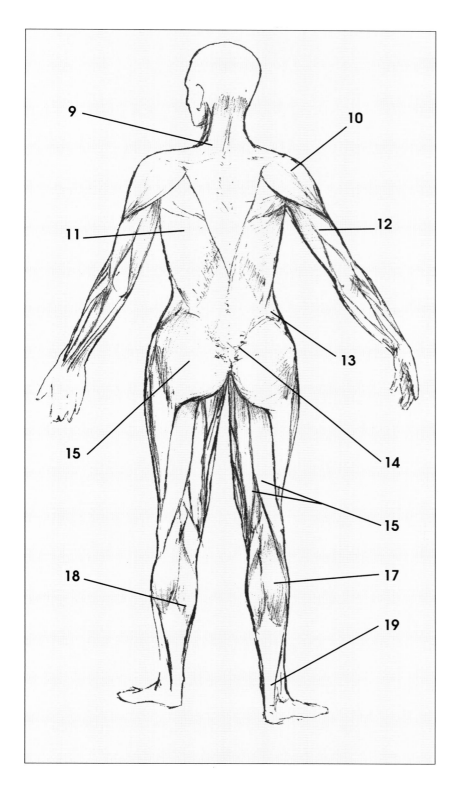

BACK VIEW

9 **Trapezius** *(holds shouder position)*

10 **Deltoid** *(moves and rotates shoulder)*

11 **Latissimus dorsi** *(moves shoulder and arm)*

12 **Triceps** *(straightens arm)*

13 **Gluteus medius** *(walking and running)*

14 *Pressure points of Sacrum (see page 24/25*

15 **Gluteus maximus** *(standing, walking, running and climbing)*

16 **Hamstrings** *(hip and knee movement)*

18 **Gastrocnemius** *(walking and running)*

18 **Soleus** *(supports leg)*

19 **Achilles tendon** *(moves foot)*

Touch + Stretch

Acknowledgements

My thanks to

The Touch and Stretch team for hard work, hassle and
fun along the way.
The models Jenny Stroud, Ginger Cowling and Britta Gartner.
Gloria Klein for permission to quote from her book "Face Up".
Special thanks to my husband Chris for believing in this book.

Carolan Evans